'This book will change how we bring up our families'
– Simon Woodroffe OBE

'A book with really helpful insights . . . we should all read
knowing that we can make a difference' – Dame Benny
Refson DBE, President of Place2Be

'Mandy is a like a surgeon for emotions. Through my
work at Big Change, I know it's easier to grow a strong
child than fix a broken adult and early prevention is key
to breaking negative cycles . . . I highly recommend this
book' – Sam Branson, co-founder of Big Change

'The book gives guidelines and positive structures that
can aid complicated, delicate and personal situations . . .
an incredibly useful source to have as a parent' – Jude Law

Proactive Parenting

Help your child conquer
self-destructive behaviours
and build self-esteem

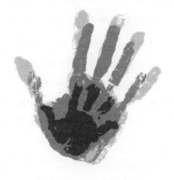

MANDY SALIGARI

First published in Great Britain in 2019 by Orion Spring
an imprint of The Orion Publishing Group Ltd
Carmelite House, 50 Victoria Embankment
London EC4Y 0DZ

An Hachette UK Company

1 3 5 7 9 10 8 6 4 2

The information contained in this book is not intended to replace
the services of trained medical professionals or to be a substitute for
medical advice and the methods may not be suitable for everyone to
follow. You are advised to consult a doctor on any matters relating to
your child's health, and in particular on any matters that may require
diagnosis or medical attention.

A CIP catalogue record for this book is
available from the British Library.

ISBN (Trade paperback) 978 1 4091 8341 9
ISBN (eBook) 978 1 4091 8342 6

Printed and bound by CPI Group (UK) Ltd, Croydon, CR0 4YY

CONTENTS

FOREWORD

As a parent, grandparent and with over twenty-four years' involvement with Place2Be, a children's mental health charity, I have often thought if I knew then what I know now, what would I have done differently? The reality is that we stand on our own shoulders of experience and it is never too late to learn and certainly never too early.

When we open our minds to learning we are exposing ourselves to the reality that there is so much we don't know and so much we have to learn. Learning is not finite; we do not arrive at a moment in time being able to say, 'we know it all'. Indeed, the more we are willing to listen and learn the more we recognise that learning is a lifelong process and one which can be enriching and exciting as well as make us feel vulnerable to the fact that we don't know it all.

Parenting is an example of this. We read books during pregnancy to prepare for birth and then more books about the different stages of our children's development, but how often do we actually admit that our own behaviour plays an enormously important role in their development and that we have much to learn at the same time as they are developing? (It is exciting to know that as individuals and as a society we can choose to open our minds to new knowledge and understanding, which will hopefully enable us to influence and enhance the futures of the children of today.)

More children and young people in the UK are struggling with their mental health than ever before. The numbers of girls under the age of eighteen being treated in hospital after self-harming has nearly doubled compared with twenty years ago and suicide rates among young people are alarmingly high. The world is rapidly changing – childhood is not what it once was, and neither is it the same for the adults; we are inundated with disturbing news and images now that we can access an overwhelming amount of information and content at the touch of a button. It can appear almost futile to ever try to keep track of the multiple different social and digital trends that seem to come and go with the seasons. Add to this the ever growing pressure to achieve, be successful, look the best, have the most friends, get the most likes etc. . . . it's no wonder that some children and young people crumble under the pressure.

While awareness and understanding of mental health has increased in recent years, services have not caught up and children and young people are waiting a long time for their initial assessment. Amid all these alarming facts and figures parents can feel at a loss about how to best protect their children and where to go when their child is in distress.

Around 50 per cent of adult mental health begins by the age of fourteen validating the importance of early intervention. Now in its twenty-fifth year, Place2Be is a charity that is built on the principle that promoting positive mental health and intervening early when problems arise can prevent mental health issues from growing and becoming more complex and entrenched. The school-based support the charity provides is very accessible and enables children, parents and teachers to ask for help without fear or stigma. It provides a safe, accessible space which aims to develop children's resilience and confidence, enabling them to have a sense of belonging and the ability to forge healthy relationships. Children, parents and teachers are reassured through access to professionally trained support, allowing them to take their fears and concerns to a stigma-free space with no lengthy waiting times and to a familiar person whose knowledge of the school environment and community provides a sense of containment thus preventing issues from spiralling out of control.

Of course, in an ideal world this type of support would be accessible to every child in every school but, partly due to budgets and partly due to the lack of suitably trained professionals, it is only a short-term solution. However, with Place2Be's knowledge, practices, clinical experience and evidence of positive outcomes, they are well based to make a significant contribution to the future mental health of the children in many more state primary, secondary and independent schools. In the meantime, parents and carers must do all they can to equip themselves with the knowledge and understanding needed to best protect their children.

Addiction is a painful experience for both the individual living with addiction and their families. We fear for our children and loved ones and we fear that our responses might cause more harm. Often, we turn our backs on the very signs that our 'gut' notices because we are frightened by not knowing how to act or what to do. There comes a moment when we realise, as parents, that perhaps we could have intervened earlier if only we had asked for help or realised that there were steps we could have taken so much sooner to build our children's self-esteem; enabling them to recognise that we are all vulnerable and that we can all develop healthy responses to that reality.

Mandy always starts with her own truth and talks from her experience of addiction and recovery and reflects throughout this most valuable book her thoughts on the underlying causes. However, at no point is blame directed towards the reader; instead in its place is a continuous, accessible explanation of the 'whys' and 'wherefores' and also, most importantly, the opportunities for prevention.

So often we read about causes and then presenting behaviours but rarely are we given advice and practical exercises which we can apply to our own parenting. As I continued to read Mandy's book several 'light bulb' moments flashed up for me and my interest in the next page or chapter never waned.

Mandy has inspired many of us when she has given her lively presentations but now she has managed to capture that energy on paper, leaving us with a sense of hope that there are ways through proactive parenting that we can actively adopt in order to enable our children to develop the life skills that will help them manage their emotions in positive ways, without resorting to destructive ones. This is a book with really helpful insights which we should all read, knowing that we can make a difference before it is too late.

Dame Benny Refson
President, Place2Be

INTRODUCTION

Many years ago, a girl in her early twenties sat on the step of an addiction treatment centre, waiting for the doors to open so she could check in. It was an agonising half hour as the urge to run argued with the knowledge that there was nowhere left to go. Rock bottom. With years behind her of challenging behaviours, a volatile school career, extreme mood swings and depressive episodes, she had sought solace in drugs and alcohol. Despite these causing her serious health consequences, including what looked like the first signs of a stroke, it was an unhappy relationship that had left her suicidal. With no more fight in her, she knew she needed help.

Twenty-eight years on, I am here to share what I have learned on my journey from middle-class England to my knees, from decades of experience of addiction recovery and as a therapist. But this is not just another recovery story: this is what I wish my parents had known, a guide for parents who want to tackle the potential of addiction in their children's lives so that they may take a different route.

Having children myself introduced me to a whole new level of vulnerability and, as I looked at their sweet faces, I knew what I wanted them to learn, what would make them resilient in this swiftly changing world. It was that which inspired me to develop a preventative model of care for parents like me, wanting to be informed so that they can take a proactive approach to bringing up their children.

The route from mild mental health symptoms, which are a normal part of growing up, into more serious issues, is an area that schools seek to address through their PSHE (Personal, Social, Health and Economic) programmes, and I am now a well-established speaker on the circuit. At first, I would only present to students, but, in line with my belief that families also deserve to be involved, I began to deliver proactive parenting talks that have become extremely popular. In turn, they have led to teacher training as, of course, teachers act *in loco parentis*. My work extended beyond addiction and into early intervention, which meant that I worked increasingly with families who would not consider their issue to be one of addiction, but who were facing difficulties with communication, asserting respectful boundaries and supporting their child to believe in themselves.

In 2008, I launched Charter Harley Street in London with long-time friend and fellow therapist Anthony McLellan. A private facility, Charter was groundbreaking in its approach, treating addiction in an outpatient setting, with a pioneering model of early intervention as its flagship programme. There was no more requirement for residential care, provided we caught people early enough. But therein lay the problem. Not the work – we were achieving success that outshone standard treatment outcomes, with people getting well rather than just getting sober – but in actually getting people to commit to treatment early enough to intervene on addiction before it got a grip. Before the devastated family relationships, the divorces, the suicide attempts, the collapsed bowel or broken bones, before the financial ruin. Because of the power of denial, the programme I had designed to literally save lives before they were lost was not an easy sell.

One of my regrets as a therapist is the stigma surrounding therapy. People seem to feel they have to be 'bad enough' before they consider it as an option. Usually someone will have tried everything before coming in – and I mean everything. One person I met had tried to kill herself six times before agreeing to commit to therapy. Thankfully, she hadn't managed it and found herself sitting opposite me instead. Over and again people arrive on their last legs – physically, mentally, emotionally, spiritually and financially crippled, seeking therapeutic help as a last resort. Of course, there are other reasons people don't access therapy sooner – long waiting lists, poor therapy options, money (as many cannot afford the commitment it takes), but also because the therapy room represents facing yourself, the very thing you seek to avoid. Bringing someone back from the brink is not easy and lots of people don't make it and that left me thinking about what could be done to bring people in at an earlier point.

My mother often used to ask me in the initial years of my recovery what else she should or could have done to intervene on my behaviour sooner. Wracked with guilt, she would ask herself over and again what she had or hadn't done, what she could have done better, what she had missed. It was painful to witness. As we talked, we always came to the same conclusion, which was that by the time it was clear that I was off the rails and needed help, I was unapproachable. Out of reach. Already gone.

This led me to thinking about what came before and how that could be conceptualised as a list of symptoms that could be addressed. I noted my past of behavioural issues like playing truant, an explosive temper, profound insecurity manifesting as defiance, neediness and swathes of time when I would just isolate. I also noted a profound distrust of authority and remembered how I used to manipulate the school counsellor to get my way, which was to slip through the net.

This, in turn, helped me see how ill-equipped my family was to effectively intervene, as many are. My parents' crime was an unhappy marriage which so very sadly affected us all as they 'stayed together for the children'. It inspired me to encourage the opportunity for all the family to get involved so that everyone has a chance to recover. This is not only in the case of addiction, I should clarify, but also in the case of any mental health disorder. It is naïve to think that the only person who suffers is the person with the diagnosis. Watching your child disappear in front of your eyes as a mental health disorder takes hold is terrifying, soul-destroying. Not least because as parents we wonder what on earth we did to cause it, knowing that we are responsible for the environment our child grows up in, but also because we think if it is our fault then maybe we can solve it, maybe we can take their pain away.

This book is aimed at you, the parent, as working with you, at any stage of a mental health diagnosis, is vital. Your feelings of fear and grief need to be understood so you can transform them from despair to useful. Your feelings of frustration and shame need to be processed so they mobilise rather than paralyse you. You need to feel that you have a grasp of what's going on, if only for yourself, so that you can stop feeling like you are constantly in the dark or, worse, contributing to the problem. It's reassuring for you as parents to feel you can help in a healthy way, and that confidence can also reassure the child. At times it can feel as if you can get nothing right and my suggestion here is to re-evaluate what you mean by the word 'right'. I talk about this in the book.

When I meet teenagers who remind me of who I was at a similar age, I feel excited at the prospect of helping them turn themselves around. It doesn't happen overnight, as it's a marathon not a sprint, but if I can work with them and crucially with their parents, we can make a big difference.

For a parent, though, to bring their child to see an addictions expert is an astonishingly brave step when a much less stigmatised label than addiction might be an option. I worked with a seventeen-year-old client who had chronic fatigue. His family was at their wits' end. He was permanently exhausted, but more powerful feelings lay beneath that were literally draining him to repress that needed to be worked through in individual and family therapy. Thanks to his courage and the willingness of his family to engage in some very difficult therapeutic work, he has gone from defeat to a bright career with an impressive university degree behind him and several years of sobriety to his credit.

Coming to see an addictions expert can feel like cracking a peanut with a mallet, especially if you don't know what you're addicted to. But in a way this is the wrong question, as it's more about how uncomfortable a person is in their skin that might cause them to use something harmful to fix themselves, to distract away. Your denial as a parent can mean that you don't spot the patterns or link the clues in time, giving addiction the opportunity to take hold right under your nose. In this book, I will make those patterns and clues quite clear and give you exercises to help you take a proactive approach. Many parents ask themselves: 'How did we end up here?' In this book, I will tell you how so you have a better chance of avoiding the pitfalls.

Working with this model will not cause any harm as it focuses on you, your child and your family so that you can feel confident of your place as a parent. It focuses on the person not on the substance, maintaining relationships rather than feeling hijacked by a behaviour or substance. It might even be so successful that you wonder why you ever went to see an addictions therapist given no addiction ever took hold!

In today's society, children are increasingly falsely empowered at younger ages to believe they know what's best for them, so they strongly challenge the parental view. Fuelled by access to the alternate parent that is the Internet and, in part, enabled by changing family structures and the ever-increasing pressure to have it all and provide the best, parents are often time-poor, leaving children to their own devices, often literally and for hours on end. Sometimes this can have devastating consequences, resulting in a child pulling further and further away from the family and out of control, and leaving the parents desperate, overwhelmed and out of their depth.

This book aims to put you back in charge. It gives you as much information as you can take on-board in ways that are easy to understand; you can then personalise your approach to parenting your own children from a positon of understanding.

What it is **not** is a guide on how to stop your child taking drugs or drinking. Instead it's about preventing mental health issues from graduating into the potentially fatal condition that is addiction. Not everyone who uses drugs and alcohol will fall foul of addiction, and this book illustrates that fact, while showing you how to be proactive in your approach to give your child the resources he or she needs to succeed.

Often people come to me saying their issue has nothing to do with addiction, choosing to work with me because I have been recommended or they have seen something that inspired them to seek me out. This is often in the case of families with a teenager they are worried about. When I first opened Charter, my teen clients and their families took up about 15 per cent of my practice. Now I'd say it is more like 75 per cent of what I do – and that's good news because in most cases, the sooner we intervene the better the outcome!

Even if you don't suffer from addiction you can benefit from the framework shown here as it's based around self-care and developing a relationship with yourself of dignity and respect.

To illustrate as best I can this shapeshifting self-destructive condition that moves like quicksilver through families, I will use stories from my own life, and from the lives of those people I've had the good fortune to work with, anonymised to preserve confidentiality. I'll provide details of what addiction looks like and what lies beneath.

It's only left for me to thank those parents whose journeys inspire this book so that other parents like them can learn to take a proactive approach to bringing up their children; so that they can put their heads on the pillow at the end of the day and think 'I have done a good enough job, just for today'.

1

COMMON EMOTIONAL PROBLEMS

I can only be as happy as my unhappiest child

As parents, we want the best for our children, and most of us will do whatever we can to try and make that happen. But sometimes no matter how hard you try, or how well you plan, life intervenes and things cause disturbance so that your plans go out of the window and you find yourself left just having to cope. Many people have issues that they know they need to manage and for which they can make plans, yet at other times problems seem to come out of nowhere. For some, life is just difficult and, at times, these difficulties are emotional or psychological.

In my view, parenting is the most important job in the world, and yet it is fraught with challenges. As you will discover in this book, it's a job where, as parents, we are always teaching and shaping our child, even when we don't intend to. Every move and every mistake has an impact. Doing a good enough job can feel impossible.

But for parents who have the additional dimension of struggling emotionally themselves, or of having a child with a mental health disorder, not only will they be doing all they can to support their child while trying to understand what is going on, but they may also have their own feelings to contend with. Alongside all the usual stresses and demands of working in family life, management of a mental health condition comes with an additional agenda of medication, doctors' appointments, a world of not knowing and often a whole new language. It's easy for parents in this position to slip into feeling hopeless and overwhelmed as they try to keep their family afloat in such uncertain and often volatile circumstances. It's tough and often I find parents have completely overlooked their own emotional needs in favour of caretaking the child.

As well as addiction, I come across many mental health difficulties in the work that I do, including anxious or depressive disorders, negative reactions to stress, borderline personality disorders, attention or behavioural disorders. What I have found brings immediate results is when I can help the person disentangle themselves from the identity of 'being' the disorder they are suffering from. This helps them to stop 'being' a problem and start 'having' one. They become people again. It can be scary, though, for people to lose the identity of a mental health label, to accept that they are separate to it. It can feel like a risk because the first thing you are likely to find is a nothingness – the absence of the mental health condition leaves an uneasy sensation, like a big yawning gap, and into that space come the feelings and they can feel sudden and disturbing. These need to be worked through so that people no longer have to be afraid of how they feel, so that they can learn to manage who they are. Of course, at times it isn't possible for people to independently manage their mental health conditions in this way, so care plans extend to include medical and psychological resources to keep them as safe as possible, but it's usually worth trying.

With any mental health condition my view is to try and help people manage as much as they can themselves, even with the short-term support of medication at the start, and then reassess the situation. Appropriately applied medication can literally be a lifesaver, but when it is used before someone is able to gain perspective independently of what's going on, or when it's over- or inappropriately used, it can block the very insight and emotional connection you need to get well.

Handling all this is stressful, in particular for young people and their families as they navigate what it is to not be 'normal' and to come to terms with their diagnosis. I also find that a great deal of emotional problems are exacerbated, if not caused, by how that person deals with stress.

Stress

Many of today's children and teenagers are under an extraordinary amount of stress, pressured to perform in today's competitive global society. But stress has become a bit of a dirty word nowadays as we are taught to avoid or blame it for our behaviour instead of seeing it as something to manage. It's become a justification for how you react, for parents and children to lose their tempers, and for not taking proper care of yourself. We know, as adults, that stress can cause damage physically and emotionally, but the pressure behind stress cannot be avoided, even by our children or teenagers. Pressure is what inevitably builds up to become stress, whether that's in the form of practical things that need to be done or in terms of expectations around e.g. money or behaviour – and it will always exist. Learning how to effectively cope with that pressure so it doesn't become damaging as stress, but perhaps motivates instead, is a vital part of becoming resilient and being able to grow up and handle the world that you live in.

For our children, however, inundated by information 24/7, there is no relief from the influence brought to them through social media and the Internet. For all the positives the global society brings, and there are many, the social downsides include a lack of anonymity, an inability to 'switch off' or take time out for Fear of Missing Out (FOMO), or of seeming odd, and the social media communication style where you are getting 'likes' one second and being humiliated or excluded another.

Nasty posts (or 'trolling') can stoke painful insecurities at a time when, in adolescent development, the sense of belonging is often already uncertain. The impact of negative attention can spread widely and quickly, alienating and scapegoating a child almost overnight. Children know this and are keen to remain 'in' with one another, placing them on high alert about what they wear, look like, weigh, their size, fashion sense or image, stimulating the part of the brain responsible for survival and which generates more stress. The list is seemingly endless, and stepping away from the family version of yourself and finding out how you fit in the world of your peers can be a terrifying stage of development for a young person. Some manage through 'Queen Bee' behaviour – a one-up bullying style designed to obscure insecurity – others may slipstream and comply or enable, and others still choose to stand out or withdraw. All to attempt to avoid the feelings of stress and fear relating to social belonging.

Life is busier, faster and more competitive than ever, and the school environment reflects this with test and teaching schedules that have timeframes all targeted towards exams: it's relentless and many of today's teens are missing the more in-depth learning in terms of a healthy consideration of themselves because they are encouraged culturally to skim the surface. This lack of focus on emotional intelligence neglects to teach them how to cope with their emotions and, more, how to make the most of them and connect with others. For some, the future seems daunting and many give up before even trying.

I believe that many children are left to their own devices far too much and do not have a parent who is there for them, in good shape themselves and able to guide and support their child emotionally as they grow up. Many parents are overstretched, often as a result of being a single-parent family or both working – as a result, the child may end up taking care of the parent or the parent sadly neglects the child's core needs, believing that to provide practical care is enough. In the absence of a parent to help them learn how to navigate their emotions, children will turn to their friends instead.

There are countless children who, when they experience profound negative emotion, will seek ways to cope with it that are self-sufficient and appear to be short-term, perhaps by hitting themselves, punching themselves, banging their head against a wall, scratching or cutting. Sometimes their families know they do this, but do not taking it seriously. It can even become a joke that the child is so sensitive. Perhaps this approach is based on the hope that it will simply go away. But in my experience these things are warning signs and should be treated seriously, as an opportunity for early intervention.

. . . .

I was working to provide information to staff at an inset day for primary school teachers. One teacher asked about a pupil, Kayla, who was seven or eight. The teacher had noticed that every time Kayla got excited it was as if she couldn't contain herself, and she was often told off for being too much or for not calming down. Kayla would often hit her hand on her desk as if, as the teacher put it, 'to use pain as a way to control excitement'. The teacher was determined to try and help Kayla manage this differently, and pro-actively to interrupt what might otherwise develop into emotional strategies that might become dangerous for Kayla.

Questions:
- What do you mean by stressed? Notice the feelings and think about what you actually need.
- Is there anything that you can do to alleviate the stress? Can you ask somebody for help? Can you organise what you have to do so it's time manageable? Can you talk it through with someone so at least you don't feel on your own?
- Are you putting unnecessary pressure on yourself? And if so, why?
- Are your feelings of stress getting in the way of your ability to do what you need to do?

Actions:
- Breathe – sit with both feet on the floor, the palms of your hands on the top of your thighs and your back straight. Soften your gaze so your surroundings are out of focus, or close your eyes. Breathe in for five counts, and out for seven. Concentrate on the wonder of your chest expanding and contracting and the feeling of breath coming in and out of your mouth or nose. Try doing this for ninety seconds three times a day.
- Go for a walk – walking mindfully (i.e. upright, at a regular stride and pace with attention on the experience of walking) is very good for managing stress, as you focus on your breath, your posture and the wonder of the mechanics of the human body as it moves. Look up and allow yourself to notice your environment.
- Be kind to yourself – the last thing you need when you're under pressure is to say or do something that makes you feel worse. Give yourself an affirmation – in the mirror if at all possible!

- Notice if what you're eating is helping you – fast foods not only have a lot of salt and sugars in them but the very nature of them encourages the pace you might be wanting to slow down! Try and eat with a friend or family member and talk while you eat, instead of eating on the run.
- Always contact your GP if you're struggling as a doctor can prescribe medication and refer you for therapy, if necessary.

Anxiety

Almost every prospective client I meet – whether parent or child – would probably describe themselves as anxious. It's a word that encompasses so many symptoms and can result positively in a person raising their game to attain a goal, or in the self-defeating overwhelm where they have little or no ability to reassure themselves or to be comforted and reassured by anyone else.

Fretting and worrying

Worrying can be a good thing as long as it doesn't get out of hand. Worrying about something can indicate that it matters to you and that you are thinking about it with some fear in an attempt to work something out. This is constructive as long as you reach the last stage and 'work something out', possibly turn what you've decided into action . . . and then let go! This is called problem-solving. But for someone who suffers from anxiety this doesn't happen, because the constant self-questioning and distrust becomes the whole process, eroding the confidence that you are capable of coming up with a good solution. Thus thoughts can go round and round about whatever is bothering you, an essay, an event or a friendship, fuelled by fear, never allowing you to get to the point of working anything out, putting any solution into action or letting go. Often people around you may get frustrated that you can't let whatever it is go or become worried themselves, leaving you embarrassed, feeling like you should hide your anxiety, which in turn makes the worry intensify as it's trapped inside you. This is quite common, for example, when children don't want to worry their parent, often because they either don't really believe their parent can help or they don't want to suffer the parent's worry themselves.

Characterised by that nagging feeling inside, when a child or teenager is over-worrying it stops them from being able to enjoy what's going on, as they check and double-check what they feel you might have forgotten, or as they wait for that feeling of dread to transform into something bad happening – which, in turn, can be a self-fulfilling prophecy. This can place demands on the parent, for example, to do things in a particular way, which can be frustrating if the anxiety doesn't then subside. Getting angry with your child, though, will make it worse, so inevitably you can become hostage to this condition too as you seek to hide your irritation.

Night-time can be the worst, when all the other practical distractions subside and the noise in your child's head can just grow. If you're asleep, they may decide not to wake you and turn to social media for support. In the early hours of the morning, some find themselves feeling desperate, with intrusive thoughts of suicide becoming more possible – that's how bad it can feel.

It's self-defeating spending time preoccupied with worst-case scenarios, and the more you think about what might happen, the worse it becomes. This might relate to the future and how everything might look hopeless or it might be related to events in the past – but it is paralysing. This is called 'projection'.

Projection

When people cannot be in the right now, in the present, they will be thinking about things in the past or the future and often torturing themselves with what might be, what has happened or what other people might think. As a result, they are profoundly distracted by thoughts which are increasingly intense, that are out of anyone's control most of the time, but that justify this anxious pattern. Additionally, the more projection you engage in, the less you are in the here and now, and the more fearful you will become about all the things you will have to face when you do eventually return to the present.

Always thinking the worst is called 'catastrophising'. For example, if your children convince themselves that they'll definitely fail an exam, be left standing alone at a party or that no one will like them, it's exhausting – they're looking ahead and seeing nothing but problems that are too big to overcome, so eventually they may just give up. But this is not necessarily the reality.

Interestingly, projection can be a way of avoiding something specific, a problem or experience that seems too difficult to face or solve at the time; then it gains a life of its own and makes it hard to face anything. Coming back into the present can feel intimidating, but it is rarely as bad as people think.

Regrets

Regrets are often a cause of anxious feelings when there's something you've said or done that you cannot forgive yourself for. Anxiousness is like a constant reminder of your guilt and fallibility, and some wear this deliberately as a kind of self-punishment, while at the same time never learning and moving on. I often think that the greatest payment or apology for something you regret is to really take on-board whatever it was you did, appreciate why, learn from it and be different next time. This is called a 'living amend'. The trouble is that when children feel regret, they will not be keen to tell their parents about it, especially as they get older, as they are likely to want to either sort it for themselves, or deny it.

In this scenario, you'll just have to wait and trust your child will work it through. Sarcastic comments or attempts to prompt your child out of this state will only serve to make it worse. I think the best approach is simply to tell your child that you can see they are suffering and to let them know you are there if only to listen.

Trauma

When a traumatic event takes place in a person's life it disturbs 'the norm', the otherwise undisturbed assumption that 'everything goes to plan'. Whatever the event, most traumas affect a sense of safety, however the trauma is handled at the time. For children this is particularly relevant as they are dependent on others to keep them safe. An experience of fear can make life seem totally unsafe and, unless it's properly addressed, that fear can take hold and develop into other anxious-type symptoms like ticking or OCD, or one of the other manifestations of addiction. Often, people who have suffered from trauma of some kind develop patterns of restlessness, foot jogging, tapping, nervous tics or patterns of behaviour that are all unconsciously designed to displace the uncomfortable feelings and almost 'burn them off'. Until the traumatic event has been properly processed it is almost impossible to remove the pervading sense of fear that colours everything in a person's life with a negative 'what if'. With so much influence around social media children are exposed to cruel social exchanges that can trigger this kind of reaction and it isn't helpful to just condemn the device or forum. Try teaching them how to manage the virtual communication style instead (see The Essentials on page 221 for more on this).

When you are anxious, you tell your brain it's right to feel fear, so your body reacts by producing adrenaline, in preparation for a threat through a flight, fight or freeze response. Flooded by this powerful chemical, in your children, appetite and sleep patterns are likely to be affected and they may report feeling sick and headachy a lot. It's exhausting for the body to keep this up and in severe cases it can cause adrenal problems that can result in glandular fever, chronic fatigue or ME (myalgic encephalomyelitis). Make sure that you pay attention to your child's self-care and see a GP and/or a therapist, if at all possible, if it looks like it's getting that serious.

Repression of thoughts and feelings

I often find that people who suffer from anxiety have stopped themselves from speaking freely, for some reason, and are frightened of what they think or feel. Instead of feeling the emotion that might come naturally, they seek to hide it, as if fearful or ashamed of even having that emotion. For example, if you are sad, then your child might be fearful of further upsetting you. If you get angry easily they may tread on eggshells around you. A longer term consequence, if this perpetuates, is that they will begin to reign in their emotions as a way of protecting both themselves and you.

Lydia came to me in her early twenties consumed with anxiousness. Exploring her childhood relationship with her mother, Lydia realised that she had not been able to feel angry with her for fear of upsetting her feelings, which she felt then would have been her responsibility to fix. Instead, she diverted these feelings of frustration and neglect into emotions that were more acceptable within her family – in her case, anxiety. She was known as anxious, but in therapy she discovered she was actually angry. Lydia had to work through a deep sense of loss around her childhood and the sense of safety that she felt she had never had to express herself honestly.

Questions:
- Trust, risk and share: talk to someone you can trust about what you're worried about, asking them first just to listen to you and not give any answers. Instead ask them to say back to you whatever it is they have heard you're worried about. Try to hear yourself.
- Write a list of what is worrying you. Beside each item write down whether you think they might be possible, likely or very unlikely or impossible. Reality check. Place the ones that are impossible or very unlikely on a list to take to a therapist if your anxiousness gets really difficult.
- If there is something you can do on your list, including asking somebody else for help, then do it. Taking help allows somebody else to give.

Actions:

- Breathe – sit with both feet on the floor, the palms of your hands on the top of your thighs and your back straight. Soften your gaze so your surroundings are out of focus, or close your eyes. Breathe in for five counts and out for seven. Concentrate on the wonder of your chest expanding and contracting and the feeling of breath coming in and out of your mouth or nose. Try doing this for ninety seconds three times a day.
- Take regular exercise – walking mindfully is very good for anxiousness as you focus on your breath, your posture and the wonder of the mechanics of the human body as it moves. Look up and allow yourself to notice your environment.
- Always contact your GP if you're struggling, as a doctor can prescribe medication and refer you for therapy.
- Take care of what you eat – sugary foods, alcohol and caffeine will make your feelings of anxiety that much worse.

Depression

A term that is used easily by many people to cover a wide spectrum of experiences, but which has at its core the common experience of persistent unhappiness, depression can be brought on by an event, a loss, negative thoughts or persistent difficulty. It can also be a result of an imbalance in your brain chemistry. Most of the time, if people feel depressed, they will seek out advice from their GPs and be put on antidepressant medications. It's worth noting that it's advisable to request therapy alongside medication so that while the antidepressants reduce the symptoms, the therapy can address the actual cause. But as people use the word to describe such a range of unhappiness, depression is an interesting presenting symptom to work with as it requires the therapist to work as a detective in a way, working with the client to uncover the origins. For some, it may be severe and connected to a chemical imbalance, perhaps where there may be a family history of depression; for others, it is a reaction to external events or emotional experiences. But what is in common in both is the negative core beliefs (like 'I am not loveable') that depression both feeds and comes out of, which makes it incredibly difficult for people suffering from it to believe that they can get well, or that it's worth getting well.

Common symptoms of depression include:

- disturbed appetite and a distinct loss or gain of weight
- disturbed sleep pattern which can translate either as extreme tiredness or inability to sleep
- feeling lethargic and lacking in energy and motivation
- loss of interest in your sex life
- feeling low, guilty, numb, hopeless, tearful and negative
- feeling agitated and irritable
- difficulty in concentrating, yet feeling preoccupied
- physical aches and pains that appear to have no physical cause

It's devastating for any parent to see your child descend into a depressive state and many parents work hard to try and motivate their child to lift their mood, but often in vain. This can then cause parents to give up or become angry, because they are afraid. The impact on the child is to continue to withdraw, often believing that this is further evidence of their own short-comings and how they can get nothing right.

Spotting genuine depression in your teen can be hard as there is often so much going on already. Teenage angst and mood swings can be just that, but they can also mask a more severe problem, and this is when it's important to listen to your gut (so make sure your gut is in good shape!). Self-care will allow you to notice when your child is struggling as you won't be distracted by your own processes. Remember, you know your child and the better your relationship with him or her, the more able you will be to help. Sometimes, it's just a case of being with the child or teen and helping them learn to tolerate the low mood, without promoting that there is an answer, as many grow through this difficult stage. For others, it is more severe. Very sadly, tragedies do happen as mental health disorders (obviously) affect the mind so your child may not be in their right mind when they make a decision. To try and avoid a tragedy, it's important that you get the proper help without abdicating responsibility to that help. I believe that if one member of the family suffers from depression, then the whole family should access support as mental health disorders affect the whole family.

In addition to the difficulty of identifying someone with genuine depression, the illness can also make a person unpredictable, so that their mood can suddenly flip from happy to raging, whether a parent or a child. In this emotional space, they can easily blame everybody else for what has gone wrong, as if they are the victim. From this impenetrable place, they glower, now ashamed, and you will not be able to reach them to comfort them. Instead, people who are depressed will often feel attacked and hopeless, even as you try to offer them help – they will struggle to receive it because of their low self-esteem. All you can do is to point out what you see and, as a parent, let your child know that you are there.

Like with anxiety, depression can also be a result of trying to repress feelings your children don't want to have, such as genuine sadness, as in the case of grief. Sometimes people would rather feel depressed than grieve, as in grieving they feel they are letting go of someone they care about.

Emotional repression is pointless and unhealthy as feelings take up space and have to go somewhere. I often tell the teens I work with that it's just not possible to hide how they feel long term as the feelings will leak out, even if it appears to be under another guise. It's also not unusual for those depressed teens to discover very lively feelings hidden away in their depression – lively feelings with sad or angry stories to tell.

Therapy is a safe place to unpack those stories and to better understand how to manage what's happened so they can choose how they file it in themselves, instead of just shutting down.

Actions:
- Try to describe how you feel without using the word 'depressed'.
- Be interested in what has happened to you, and think about what you would like to take from that experience. What can you learn?

- Allow people to identify with you – you're not alone – and to help you. Let go of the sanctuary of depression.
- What's your 'stinking thinking' that sets you up to see things negatively?
- What negative thoughts do you have about yourself? Are they really true? And is it fair to say these things about yourself? Do they have to be true?
- Go for a walk – walking mindfully works well to shift depression as you focus on your breath, your posture and the wonder of the mechanics of the human body as it moves. Look up and allow yourself to notice your environment.
- Be kind to yourself – the last thing you need when you're under pressure is to say or do something that makes you feel worse. Give yourself a positive affirmation – in the mirror if possible!
- Notice if what you're eating is helping you – putting healthy food into your body is kind and esteeming and will totally challenge your depression because you are showing yourself that you matter by treating yourself with care.
- Always contact your GP if you're struggling as a doctor can prescribe medication and refer you for therapy, if needed. EMDR therapy might help (see The Essentials on page 221).

Attention deficit disorders (ADD and ADHD)

The classic (negative) symptoms of ADD (Attention Deficit Disorder) or ADHD (the 'H' refers to the hyperactivity dimension of the disorder) are impulsivity, difficulty concentrating and agitation, which means that sufferers often underachieve at school, where they can be labelled as disruptive or lazy; in work, where they can be experienced as inconsistent despite moments of brilliance; and in relationships, where their mood swings can become intolerable to the other person. Projects get started with huge enthusiasm and then remain unfinished. Plans are made but not followed through with good organisation or time management. Repeated patterns of negative behaviours mean that nothing appears to change and lessons don't appear to be learned, which fuels feelings of disappointment in relationships. Further impulsivity and poor organisational skills make it difficult to manage money, emotions and more complicated social dynamics like relationships and family life.

All this can obviously have a big knock-on effect on how people feel about themselves, and all these difficulties can profoundly damage self-esteem. This is despite the upsides to this kind of mood disorder, whereby people are often very creative and original in their thinking, or engaging and generous to be around – all of which is easily overlooked. It's difficult for someone with ADD or ADHD to work within the system that exists in society, as it can feel quite rigid and demanding, so much so that their sense of belonging and belief that they fit can be compromised.

It's tough for parents too, as they wrestle to manage their own feelings, when witnessing their child 'going off on one', as one parent described it, adding the child was 'too painfully close to normal'.

There is no hard and fast evidence as to where ADD comes from, but it seems to run in families. The environment is, of course, also an influence, including the baby's experience in pregnancy and at birth, food allergies and interestingly overstimulation, including excessive use of television and video games.

Questions:
- Do you notice that your child struggles to start an activity or, once started, to complete it?
- Or that he/she fidgets a lot and seems to struggle with concentration?
- Or that he/she seems to be drawn to high-intensity or dangerous activities?
- How does that make you feel?

Actions:
- Try to notice what he/she is good at intuitively and remember to see the good in this.
- Use a meditation CD or technique to help your child learn how to self-soothe or calm down.

- Limit time spent on screens and take regular breaks to run around or play with a ball or ride a bike – it's an important physical counterbalance to the overstimulated brain.
- Try to encourage creative activities as well as physical ones – this is about learning how to channel excess energy effectively.
- Notice if what you're all eating is helping or exacerbating issues. Avoid fast foods or ready meals and try to eat fresh food with low-sugar content.
- Always contact your GP if you're struggling as a doctor can prescribe medication and refer you or your child for therapy, if necessary.

Growing up in the twenty-first century is stressful enough as our children navigate the fast-moving communication constructs that dictate their world. It's stressful for parents too, as we can feel ever more deskilled or afraid in this fast-paced environment, while trying to guide and support with authority. For time-poor parents, the opportunity to connect and decompress by talking things through continues to reduce. This creates a build-up of pressure and stress that can easily convert into symptoms that might be recognised as any one of the mental health disorders described here.

Suffering from any of these mental health conditions can feel hopeless and paralysing because of how awful it is to have your mind, body and feelings in civil war. Being around somebody in this state, even if they are pretending to be OK and trying their best to contain their symptoms, can feel frightening too, like walking in a minefield. At any moment, you can inadvertently trigger an explosion that results in somebody getting hurt, and usually without warning.

Spotting that something is wrong takes courage because it's the first step to doing something about it. I don't want to encourage parents to engage in knee-jerk reactions as a result of reading this because many children will present with many of these symptoms that I will describe in this book, but they will grow out of them, and the negative symptoms will pass. But if the symptoms persist or if there is a pattern to the symptoms, then it's important not to ignore them. Doing nothing is worse than doing something and the proactive position is to honestly assess what's going on and to take responsibility for your decisions. Even if you decide to do nothing, as long as it's a conscious decision, you are, in fact, doing something!

It's worth mentioning that a sign of a healthy relationship is when children tell their parents what's going on, how happy they are, as well as how unhappy, but the parent has got to remember the context. Childhood and teendom are intense times – emotions are felt keenly, slights hit home deeply and passions run high. It's vital to listen, but not to overreact, and yet it's important to take action when necessary. Being able to do this will be easier if you, the parent, are in good shape yourself.

How to spot it if I need to take action

Listen carefully to the one-off experiences but be aware of any emerging patterns of behaviour, as it's the patterns that really paint the picture. Many parents will not react or intervene, even if their child is often getting drunk, for example, as they will put it down to the company their son or daughter is keeping and seek to alter that, instead of looking at their child's relationship with alcohol. If they are getting drunk then they are the ones who are drinking – that might seem simple enough, but it's interesting how often this kind of sign is missed and the right questions are not asked.

Not talking, withdrawing and seeming to isolate, an increase in anxiety or a presence of low mood or depression are worth noting, as are extreme changes in behaviour or mood. Sometimes a child will present with something more tangible as a way of asking for help, like in a difficulty in sleeping or change in appetite or in unexplainable aches and pains. If this is what's happening, listen to your child, at the same time as asking yourself why they don't simply tell you what's going on. See if you can make changes to make yourself more approachable or available to them.

Trust your gut, talk to your child, your partner and other parents to see if you might be onto something or if you are overreacting because of your *own* anxiousness or stress. See if there is anything you can do to help ease the situation, even just a little at a time. The pain I often witness is in parents who ignored their gut instinct.

Unsupported, sufferers of poor mental health and their families struggle on, trying to cope with the difficulties of everyday life as they watch 'everybody else' seemingly have it so easy. This can be in a pattern of compare and despair: if you compare how you feel against how everybody else looks, you are likely to be left coming off worse.

Poor mental health doesn't only affect the sufferer: it affects everybody around them. When you start to feel that this is just your lot in life and that you cannot fix your or your loved one's mental health problems, perhaps that you can't even keep them at bay, then you may turn to patterns of self-medication either to take the pain away or to provide temporary relief. Pivotal in the self-destructive behaviours people use to either attempt to cope, escape or belong – this pattern of self-medication is called 'addiction', a mental health condition in it's own right.

2

WHAT IS ADDICTION?

Emotions are what we have the most of and know the least about: handle them or they will handle you

My working definition:

'Addiction is the *mismanagement of your emotion* by *using something outside of yourself, repeatedly,* in an attempt to *fix how you feel* to the *detriment* of yourself'

Using this model, at times it might feel like you are pathologising 'normal behaviours', seeing the potential for addiction in everything. I'm not trying to create a false epidemic, but you should also recognise that denial is lethal. I meet so many people who wish they had listened to their gut instincts earlier so I encourage you to not ignore yours. If addiction is developing in someone you love it will start in warped reactions or in the common mental health conditions touched on in Chapter 1. But it's in these behaviours I am hoping to give you the confidence to intervene.

The stats have never been good around addiction recovery; despite ambitious claims by treatment centres, the widely held view behind the scenes remains 3: 3: 3 (so, a third recover, a third relapse and a third die of addiction). This is because rehabs tend to treat the symptoms, i.e. the manifestation of the addiction – that is, the substance, and not the person. In part, this is due to time and limited resources, but it's also because, as parents and people, we often wait until the symptom is so extreme that it demands attention as a priority. Before that there is often a long list of doctors' appointments and medical diagnoses of anxiety disorders, depression, mood disorders and the medication to go with it, but with no real solution achieved. As all treatment centres know, it's appropriate to treat what will kill you first – for an alcoholic that's alcohol, not the low self-esteem that drove that person to drink in an addictive manner in the first place. Thus in doing this, often the roots of the illness remain unaddressed.

The term 'addict' remains one that is loaded with stigma and viewed with prejudice, seen by many as a sign of weakness or self-indulgence, and measured in terms of how much a 'drug of choice' is used and the pursuant disturbance to behaviour. I have had clients who would prefer to be labelled bipolar and be on lithium for the rest of their life (a drug that can damage the kidneys and the thyroid), rather than accept the term 'addict'. All you have to do to be in recovery from addiction is stop using, and practise good self-care, but this is so much harder than it sounds for someone who is in self-loathing. If only therapy were offered first. It is my frequent experience that once the client has dealt with the original trauma, the medication can be vastly reduced or they can come off it completely. I am not diminishing the value of medication, but challenging its status as the best, first and often only option.

This is a political issue as much as anything – of course money is made through the pharmaceuticals, liability is contained through box ticking, and therapy waiting lists are long, with therapist skill varying widely. But recovery from addiction is a personal journey and one that is completely possible and very rewarding in every sense, but it is an area hugely under-resourced and that is a genuine social tragedy.

Rather than a weakness of character, I see addiction as a way that people might avoid being vulnerable, even if what they 'use' causes harm. Thus the physical manifestations of addiction, such as drugs, alcohol or self-harming behaviours, are usually symptoms of the emotional wounds people may have experienced at some point in their lives. And to be clear, it is not just the existence of a trauma or a disturbing event that can cause these emotional wounds, far more it is how they are handled at the time or how they are remembered that can cause the problem. If, for example, a person experiences a stressful or frightening event but comes out safely or is affirmed in relation to that experience, they are likely to build confidence.

But if that same person was told that they nearly died, it was their fault or the negative potential of the situation is reinforced, then they might emerge from the experience with the deeply isolating emotion of fear.

This plays directly into how addiction is perceived and misunderstood, so that hidden in plain view it continues to destroy families and run rampant, virtually unchecked, through the very fabric of our society. Of course, you can become addicted to an addictive substance, or drug of choice, but that is just the tip of the iceberg; a physical addiction. The pathological addiction comes in people not in packages, and I'm not talking about an 'addictive personality', I'm talking about somebody changed by something that happened or by an environmental influence that means they live their life avoiding connection, avoiding being vulnerable. It is not about the drugs or how much you use. It is not about the alcohol or whether or not you drink in the morning. It is about you and me. It's about your relationship with yourself, and to successfully treat it we need to focus in the most effective place.

My working definition (on page 25) is useful not only because it signposts how to spot the addictive process developing, but also when it is broken down (as follows) as it shows where the work needs to be done to treat, or more importantly to prevent the onset of this life-threatening condition.

1. Mismanagement of emotion

Feelings are what we have the most of but know the least about. They influence so much of what we do and yet often we seek to deny or alter them. If the culture within your family is to try to promote a particular feeling or repress another, then your child will never understand in their own right what that feeling is and how to manage it, learning instead from the example you set. It is interesting to note that many people who suffer from addiction report extreme experiences of anger in childhood. Extreme in that either they have witnessed violence that causes them to fear anger or passive aggression that denies the existence of anger and which can cause a child to feel ashamed of having this primal emotion. Many people seeking therapy, and especially for addiction, have to learn how to effectively handle their anger in a healthy way. When you mismanage your emotion, you don't handle it well, maybe displacing it onto something or someone else, by repressing or denying it, maybe by having feelings about having feelings – e.g. feeling ashamed about feeling angry, or angry about feeling vulnerable. In order to manage your emotion well, you need to first accept that emotions are a normal part of healthy living and not deny any of them, instead learn how to have them in a manageable and respectful way

2. Using something outside of yourself

This needs to prompt you to notice if your child has a pattern of using something to fix or displace onto, when they experience feelings they don't know what to do with. Do they use screens as a way to avoid or displace anger? Do they cruise the cupboards for food when they feel bored? Do they smoke when they feel vulnerable? Or have a drink when they feel fear? – Or do you? It might be useful to notice your own external props while you're observing theirs, the things to which you turn when you struggle with a feeling or an experience.

In the next chapter, you will find fifteen manifestations of addiction™ which I have collated into a list and which are the most common 'addictions' your child might adopt, ones you or they can go to rehab to get treatment for. To explain, there is nothing more normal than putting up an umbrella when it rains to protect you from getting wet, but if you then keep that umbrella up just in case it rains, you will miss the sunshine. In the same way, if, after a long day at work, you find having a drink or eating some comforting food is a pleasure, making you feel better and helping you to relax then I have no quibble with that. But if, as a result of having that drink, you have another and another, and you go on to behave in a way that you know you will regret, even if you don't care to openly admit it, then that might signal a problem. Or even if, in anticipation of having that well-deserved drink or treat, you are impatient with the needs of those who depend on you, like your children, as they become an obstruction to what you want, again there is more to this drinking than pleasure. Put simply, for parent or child: **if your coping mechanism causes trouble, then it is trouble.**

It is common for parents who come in for advice about their children to discover that their own dependence on alcohol or maybe food drives some of their difficulties with their children – they may try to over-organise their children, rush them or shout at them in their urgency to clock off (or have a drink), and the children may react badly to being shouted at, especially if they think it's unfair. But these parents would not usually call themselves 'alcoholic'.

3. Repeatedly

Do you do the same thing over and again to attempt to cope, in relation to a certain feeling or event, without really considering if it is helping or not? One of the forms of 'insanity', as is understood in step 2 of the Twelve Steps Fellowship Programme (see The Essentials on page 221) is that people who suffer from addiction will do the same thing over and again, and yet expect a different result. It's as much about how the person who eats a few biscuits and then feels sick, saying they don't understand why they just did that, will do it again, as the alcoholic, who after a binge swears to go teetotal, a gambler after a flutter promises their wife that's the last time or a sex addict, distraught in their apology when they are found out, swears fidelity forever. But experience tells me that if that action is your emotional coping mechanism, you will do it again, even though the backlash from it hurts you. So what we need to teach is how to note the consequences and learn from them, play the tape forward, alongside recognising and respecting your emotions, so that you can find different ways to react and the time to do it.

You might be surprised how resistant people are – even if they have sought my advice, even if they are on their knees – to accept that their way doesn't work. But to surrender to help is a necessary step and it can be the most painful, as it involves the intimacy of being seen and it can feel humiliating for some to accept help.

4. To fix how you feel

Why fix feelings? The desire to fix a feeling or emotion is often driven by a lack of acceptance of that feeling – like telling someone not to be angry or sad when perhaps being angry or sad is actually the most natural and healthy response to whatever has happened. Emotions are natural and learning how to have them all in a healthy way is essential for a balanced emotional life. Further, the idea that feelings need to be fixed, got rid of, repressed or even the idea that you need to 'get the feelings out' implies that they do not belong as part of you. This thinking invites a purge process, suggesting that some feelings shouldn't exist or are wrong.

In fact, a healthy person will digest their experience, and have access to a full repertoire of emotion from sadness and fear, through healthy shame and anger and into happiness and all the variations of these feelings throughout, but they will have them without repeatedly hurting themselves or those who care about them. This can only happen if a person has had the opportunity to experience the feelings safely, respecting them and learning how to express and regulate them. Without practice most things are difficult, and that includes managing your feelings, which I believe takes a lifetime to master, so we need to start young.

Learning how to tolerate feelings is not as simple as just saying 'sit with your feelings' either. It is about being curious about how you feel as part of your investment in yourself as someone you will spend the rest of your life with. Noticing the feelings rather than trying to change them or trying to change the circumstances can open up a whole new world of understanding which can lead to profound tolerance and acceptance.

5. To the detriment of yourself

If you stop and evaluate what it is you turn to when you are feeling a certain way, you can evaluate if that 'fix' is helping you or somehow causing you hurt or pain. Certainly drinking heavily or taking drugs, cutting yourself or starving yourself to cope with anger or stress are obvious self-destructive patterns of 'coping', but even in subtler forms the 'harm' is the disbelief that you can cope with your own emotions so you delegate the emotional process onto something else, and over time this will lower self-confidence and damage self-esteem.

One very important question is: does your coping mechanism cause you harm, trouble or pain? If it does, then it's worth looking at and starting to explore different ways to cope or respond to life's stimuli. All the people who I have worked with over the many years I have been a therapist have initially sought solace, relief or even courage from their drug of choice only to discover that they suffer more from the coping mechanism than from the original hurt. There is a saying that goes 'you hurt me, so I hurt me', and there is real truth in that. One way that people try to control feeling hurt by others, or by something over which they have no control, is to take back the control by hurting themselves. This is an example of automatic behaviour – they might seem conscious of what they are doing but they are not. They are simply playing out an inevitable pattern that has already been practised and established in their mind as a response.

It is also very common for people who suffer from addiction to believe that they are only hurting themselves, not anybody else, and so they are irritated by family members feeling upset or worried about them because it inhibits their right to treat themselves as an 'island'. I don't believe anybody is an island but rather that we are all interconnected and that it is quite normal to care and be cared for. One of our core social motives as human beings is that of belonging, and this comes from connecting with other people. I actually believe the core of the addictive process lies in abandonment of self through fear of being vulnerable which means the addict isolates. In its simplest form, learning how to connect as an equal, without being better than the other or placing yourself at somebody else's feet, is the key to recovery and therefore implicit in any effective prevention model.

Detriment to self can be measured in physical terms such as in the plight of the alcoholic, the drug addict, the anorexic or the self-harmer. The damage is physical and visible and measurable. Likewise, for the gambler the damage is financial. Or for the sex and love addict the consequences are broken relationships. But the damage that kills from behind the façade of functional lives, the damage that makes group therapy so magical when all the different forms of addiction sit in a room together and begin to identify despite their differences, that damage is in the relationship with yourself. Within that identification we find the answers for prevention: **if you genuinely care about yourself you will find it hard to harm yourself in any way.**

1.

The child, between nought to six years old, is in the early stages of development and is most vulnerable to the influences around them

2.

People-pleasing

An experience or their environment terrifies them without sufficient reassurance, so they defend against feeling vulnerable and out of control by pretending to be someone else, a 'good' girl or boy, and people pleasing (crucially trying to *control* what others think of them)

3.

Overachieving
People-pleasing

This works, so others think they know the child as e.g. 'good', which the child experiences as both a pressure to continue to be good and as lonely, as they feel a fraud. As a result, they add another version of themselves in case they can't keep up being 'good', like overachieving

4.

Overachieving
People-pleasing
Shame   Isolation
Fear

When others respond to these 'false versions' of the child, the child can feel ashamed and afraid of being found out as a 'fraud'. They begin to believe that they *are* the problem and become heavily invested in not letting anyone see who they 'really' are

5.

Self-harm
Overachieving
People-pleasing

This can create anxious symptoms that the child might try to deal with through behaviours, such as self-harming, to help alleviate the tension they feel of self-hatred and being a fraud, and to express the anger they'd rather deny.

In using self-harm, they have to be willing to believe they are the problem, with a shame-based core belief like 'I am not loveable', 'I am not good enough' or 'I am wrong'. These beliefs make it OK to hurt themselves, therefore 'crossing their vulnerable selves out'.

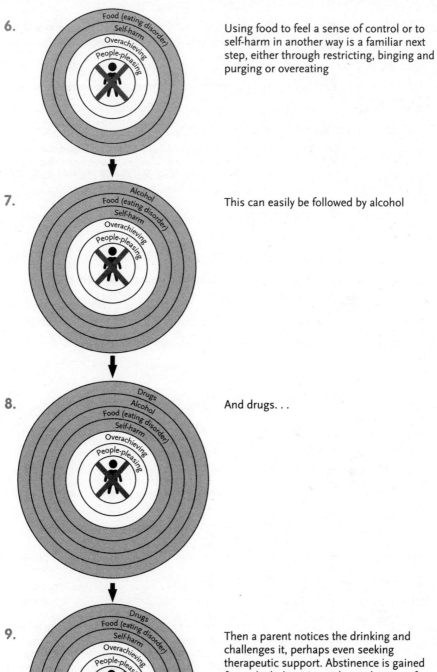

6.

Using food to feel a sense of control or to self-harm in another way is a familiar next step, either through restricting, binging and purging or overeating

7.

This can easily be followed by alcohol

8.

And drugs. . .

9.

Then a parent notices the drinking and challenges it, perhaps even seeking therapeutic support. Abstinence is gained from alcohol or it's vastly cut down . . . for a while. There is an inevitable relapse since by removing the alcohol only one of the layers of defence has been removed or challenged. I believe this is why addiction is considered a 'chronic relapsing condition'.

Until the original experience of vulnerability is addressed and the person helped to be comfortable in their own skin, I believe they will continue to seek to avoid and self-medicate. An important part of effective treatment is to learn how to treat yourself with curiosity, kindness and boundaries. Therefore, a vital part of prevention is in the parenting, so you teach curiosity, kindness and boundaries from the outset. This can be done best when it's how you also treat yourself (and others). One begets the other.

The diagram on pages 32–3 shows the way a child who feels extreme fear around their sense of vulnerability (usually between nought and six years old, prior to development of cognitive ability) compensates by putting behaviour in place to manage their feelings of extreme sensitivity (i.e. develops an addictive process). This child will look like any other child, but for them the compensating behaviour is doing something different. It is making them feel safe or experience a sense of belonging; it is setting up a pattern of looking outside of oneself for resources that should be developed internally. This child will (as above) be a 'good girl' to please, feel that 'good' isn't 'good enough' and so persists in seeking increasingly perfect behaviour in herself. This may result in a private and self-destructive pattern to release tension (such as self-harm), which frequently graduates into an eating disorder. Once the eating disorder is on-board, it does what all the other types of compensating do and takes over.

This pattern of development means that the person has been reliant on resources outside of themselves in an attempt to cope with their emotions; when you take those things away, the person is usually exposed at the age they were when they started compensating. Thus, the therapeutic work is to re-parent. To help someone grow up and develop the internal resources while preventing them from self-defeating 'shortcuts'.

Where does addiction come from?

I'm often asked where I think addiction comes from and I believe the following to be the most significant influences in developing addiction so that it is genetically influenced rather than determined:

1. Family predisposition
2. Neurological influence
3. Traumatic event and how that's responded to
4. Family and social environment

1. Family predisposition

In the discussion of 'nature vs nurture', this one comes under both. What I mean by family predisposition is the culture within the family, particularly in relation to emotional expression. Lots of people ask me if I believe that addiction is genetically passed through families, but I don't believe there is any evidence to support this. However what is interesting is that through self-report many families with a classic 'addict' in their midst come from families of addiction (or of extreme disturbance around The Core Characteristics™, which you can read about in Chapter 4). What is clear is that addiction begets addiction (but does that mean that pattern can apply to recovery, too?).

2. Neurological influence

Another 'nature' influence, here I am referring to what might be described as the baby's inherent personality, their neurological make up, born of their genes and their experience in the womb and of birth. So often I hear reports from parents as they wring their hands in despair, feeling like they no longer know their teenage son or daughter, that as a child they were difficult, or 'oversensitive'. It's as if the problems reach all the way back to those first months and years, with the parent feeling ever more redundant and deskilled and the child seemingly predetermined to be difficult in some way. But the environment in early life (nought to six) has a huge influence on brain and personality development, and I struggle to believe that a child is simply born difficult.

3. Traumatic event and how that's responded to

When something happens in somebody's life to disturb their sense of safety they will compensate (think umbrella in the rain principle). But not all rauma causes addiction. Many people experience traumatic events such as divorces, personal loss or assault, to name only three, and don't develop addiction, and this interests me. What is it that happens or doesn't happen to cause a difference? I believe this difference exists in the containment or reaction around that traumatic event at the time. Perhaps we can gain important insight on this from PTSD – post-traumatic stress disorder. It is the stress following a trauma, the lack of the effective self-soothing that allows the person to recalibrate back into their skin and into a safe sense of self that is so symptomatic of this disturbing disorder. So perhaps it is not the event itself that is the significant factor in the development of addiction, perhaps it is how that event is handled, which again puts power into the hands of those around the troubled individual to make a difference.

. . . .

A friend of mine, who is a therapist, had a car accident where she rolled her car with two of her children inside. As soon as the car came to a halt, she started the process of containing the trauma, seeking to reassure and prevent any knock-on effect of the shock. She gave a reality check, describing precisely what had happened with no exaggeration or minimisation and encouraged both her children to breathe and shake off the trauma, asserting themselves back into the 'now', once they were safely on the side of the road, to recalibrate back into their bodies. None of them had been physically hurt but all of them were shaken and it is that 'shaken' that she had sought to address immediately. A policeman arrived on the scene and as he approached her and her children he had started to say how lucky they were because . . . she stopped him in his tracks, taking him to one side to ask what he was about to say. He had been about to say how lucky they were that X, Y and Z hadn't happened (e.g. a car or lorry coming in the opposite direction on the blind corner). She told me later that she had felt a flush of anger at his lack of trauma training that meant his clumsy words could have put into her children's minds the notion of 'what if' at a time when they were open by being so shaken up. A natural reaction to express relief at a time when there is shock, but it is a natural reaction that can be significant in causing PTSD symptoms that can haunt people long after the incident has passed. Thankfully, on this occasion my friend managed to intervene, and I get the impression the policeman got the sharp side of her tongue as she was protective in her own shocked state!

None of us can change what has happened to someone but we can absolutely help them 'file it' in such a way that it causes no further trouble, or reduces that consequence. The ability to hold, reassure, reality check, comfort and make somebody feel safe comes from the ability to do that for yourself. Again this reinforces the need for a parent to practise good self-care so that they can be calm and reassuring in the face of life's difficult events which happen to us all.

4. Family and social environment

Who we are and how we connect is what we learn in our social groups, the first of which is the family. We try out behaviours, we adopt roles, we observe other people's behaviour and their roles and we learn how and who to be in the world.

It's so interesting when I meet people who have a parent or parents who are alcoholic and yet that person also drinks or gravitates to someone who does. You'd think they would avoid it as a result of growing up with those vivid negative experiences, but more often than not instead they will follow suit.

* *

Trish came to see me again several years after completing a period of therapy with me. She had met the 'man of her dreams' and got married, having a child two years into their marriage, at which point her husband had started drinking. When Trish had met him he had barely drunk at all and so she was bewildered by his swift decline into what she could only describe as alcoholism. Given her own father's alcoholism, it didn't surprise me that she had chosen a similar profile in her husband because Trish had

never really come to terms with the man her father actually was,
holding onto her fantasy instead. Trish insisted that she hadn't
known that her husband had the potential to be a drinker because
of his virtually teetotal state when they met, but as we worked
together, it became clear that the parallels between him and her
father went far beyond the alcohol and that something in her
less conscious mind had found him familiar. Attracted by this
familiarity, Trish had interpreted it as love. Her move to attend
therapy at this point allowed Trish not only to work through this
insight but also to parent differently, accepting her own child-
hood experience as the child of an alcoholic.

It is my personal belief that we are set up in childhood to be primed to gravitate towards certain people, places and things as a result of our family and social environment and that it is only when we become acutely conscious of these influences that we are put in a position of (potential) 'free will', whereby we can actually make a free decision for ourselves. But it takes enormous self-discipline to challenge this kind of priming whereby I would almost say that you could otherwise hit your teens, press 'play' and the rest is inevitable.

The family is the greenhouse within which we are grown from seed to seedling to plant, transferring ourselves outside when we become trees. And in that greenhouse atmosphere we are shaped. As parents, we are the gardeners, teaching all the time. Not just when we decide to tell a child something, to uphold the rule or to reward, but in all that we do and how we are. Especially before the child turns six or seven, when the frontal cortex becomes the primary filter through which they experience life, the child is simply soaking up an atmosphere like blotting paper in water and that water is us as parents and the environment that we create for our children 24/7. It is where the child learns about communication, attachment in relationship, identity and sense of worth in the world. For this important job there is little guide beyond what our own parents did or didn't do. The key is to learn from your own childhood and forgive so that as far as possible you are free to be independent of your priming.

Tenka came to see me for help with her relationship with her son who had quite literally stopped talking to her. She was distraught and described how when she had given birth, she had promised her son he would never feel as lonely or rejected as she had throughout her childhood. Somehow as a result she seemed to have suffocated her child with all the love she wished she had had, causing him to reject her so that the pattern was repeated, and she felt rejected and lonely. She had come to talk about her son, but the work Tenka needed to do was in relation to her own childhood experience. Her son's withdrawal had been a healthy reaction, cruel as it seemed, as he could not be the solution to her childhood pain.

Addiction is a mental health condition that takes hold around how you feel about yourself and therefore how you behave towards yourself and others. It's a condition that affects your mind, your body, your emotions and your soul so that you are increasingly consumed by negative thoughts, with a busy and obsessive mind; you stop taking care of your most basic needs around health, hygiene, food and sleep; you warp and avoid your emotions so that they compel you into irrational behaviours; you displace your own unresolved experiences onto others and then feel disappointed when you still feel hurt; you lose faith, love, gratitude and hope, and you are increasingly alone.

In the anonymous fellowship rooms across the world addiction is known as 'a hole in the soul' and, in that description, we must find not only where the focus should be to recover, but how to prevent this parasitic predator that is addiction. We must challenge our own fear and prejudice as parents and recognise our children's need to self-medicate if for whatever reason we have not been there for them in a way that has been helpful and supportive. It is time for us to embrace our responsibility and to treat parenting as the most important job there is.

Questions:

- How do I feel around others' anger, fear or sadness?
- Do I seek to take these feelings away, to explain them away or fix them, if my child feels them? (E.g. 'don't be angry'.)
- If so, why is that?
- How do I express my own anger, fear and sadness?
- Do I ever 'use' anything to cope with these feelings?
- Is there a downside to this?
- What have I learned? (E.g. that I am afraid of my child feeling fear.)

3

THE MANIFESTATIONS
OF ADDICTION

If the drug of choice is the problem, then I am not an addict

Whenever I mention addiction, people automatically think of drugs and alcohol, as if they are the only types. They are not. They are simply two of fifteen manifestations of this relational condition, which is often fostered in childhood and then reinforced through life experience.

As an openly recovering addict, I am often asked what I was addicted to, as if that is a natural question to ask with an easy answer. And, although I'm happy to explain my addiction story, and no longer feel shame about my journey in life, I also don't want to mislead people by answering as if the question is a valid one.

As I have already said in Chapter 2, addiction comes in people not in packages like drugs or alcohol – perhaps the more appropriate question is: 'what happened to you that made you want to hurt yourself that much?' Admittedly, some drugs are addictive by the nature of their composition and create a physical craving in the person using them. This never really goes away because the alternate state of the experience is the escape most addicts seek, even if that state is actually more negative. It is the psychological and emotional craving for escape and relief that really drives an addiction, and until we focus on this as a priority by being proactive rather than waiting for the addictive process to establish itself, addiction will remain a chronic relapsing condition.

Sobriety should be the means to a sustainable recovery not the goal in and of itself. As a priority, it's vital to get your child or yourself sober from whatever is being used to self-medicate, because it's probably causing harm, but as importantly because it will block you from connecting with yourself or your loved one and from developing compassionate insight, which is when the proper can work begin. For as long as you are using whatever your drug of choice is, you are not available to be reached – FULL STOP!

When I talk about addiction, I am talking about a person's resistance, *profound* resistance to being vulnerable so that they compensate and avoid being known, even in ways that cause them harm.

In my view, there are now fifteen common ways people do this and I have created a list that I believe to be useful. I acknowledge that this list provides a brief departure from the Diagnostic and Statistical Manual of Mental Disorders (DSM–5, published by the American Psychiatric Association), which is widely recognised by health professionals and government bodies as the clinical guideline for diagnosis and treatment of mental health disorders. However, this departure does not disagree with these guidelines; it adds to them. I have worked with addiction over the last twenty years and this list includes habits and behaviours for which you can be admitted into traditional rehab anywhere in the world to get clean, sober and achieve healthy bottom lines or abstinence. Often people report trying to control food or starting to smoke in childhood as a way of managing how they feel or others might become people-pleasers or rescuers (codependency) for the same reason. Whatever the 'drug of choice', any overuse of the following to fix feelings should send up warning signs to you, particularly if a pattern begins to emerge:

1. Drugs-prescription, legal, illegal

If you want to know about drugs, what they do, what the dangers are and any other factual information, your best place to look is the Frank website (www.talktofrank.com). This is dedicated to providing up-to-date information on the ever-changing, ever evolving selection of drugs available. Please don't think that because of your postcode, affluence, education, bravado or environment that you will prevent your child from running into drugs. They are easy to get hold of, many can be bought online with pocket money and delivered to the door at home. In my view, they are commonplace and almost taken for granted as part of the teenage experience. I would almost dare to say that all teenagers are in social environments where they are offered drugs and may take them, at least once.

Drugs generally fall into one of three categories: hallucinogens, opiates and stimulants, and come in different forms of drugs that you can smoke, snort, inject, inhale, take as a pill – and many teenagers will manage a cocktail of drugs in order to manage their moods, energy levels, capacity to drink, sleep, sexual activity and to control their appetite. Word spreads more quickly today among the teen population through social media, thus normalising the use of drugs and encouraging experimentation.

The whole 'drugs are bad' approach, which is fear-based, is quickly dismissed in the face of personal experience. As a parent, I would prefer my children do not take drugs, but if they do try them, I want them to take them safely.

2. Alcohol

This is such an established part of Western culture that it is often overlooked as a genuine problem, even when somebody is regularly displaying what I would recognise as symptoms of alcoholism. The stigma around admitting you are an alcoholic, or associated with displaying signs of alcoholism, is so strong, perhaps because 'everybody drinks', so the shame is greater if trouble always follows when you drink. I think it's also very scary to consider that you are dependent on alcohol because it is widely recognised now that abstinence is a necessary part of effective treatment through the Twelve Steps approach as advocated by Alcoholics Anonymous (AA).

Every day, I hear resistance about going to AA. People say 'I am not like those people', as if everybody in those rooms is some kind of a loser. That is not my experience of AA. Some of the most extraordinarily creative, sensitive, successful and clever people are among those I have met in those rooms.

The prejudice around drinking, the pride in being able to 'put a lot away', the fear of what life might be like sober, all delay people's access to proper help. For me, this is a very real social tragedy. More than that there is almost a badge of pride in social groups around how much you can drink, reinforced by drinking games and the often reckless, uninhibited experiences that happen under the influence.

Don't misunderstand me for being a member of the anti-fun squad: I love a good time as much as anyone. I just happen to have borne witness to the casualties from addiction and I bring those to you in the hope of educating and counterbalancing popular view.

3. Food – anorexia, bulimia, overeating

I have focused on the above three main experiences of an eating disorder, but there are others, such as orthorexia (obsessive healthy eating). Not everyone in the medical profession or in the field of therapy and health-care would agree that eating disorders fall within the spectrum of an addiction and some seriously oppose this way of thinking. For me, what works works, and I have history of successfully treating people with eating disorders through the addiction model that I work with. Therefore, I include them in my list.

I should note that there are schools of thought that would consider sugar as an addictive substance, and I would agree that most of my clients have a relationship with sugar that they are barely aware of and that causes them negative consequences. For example, an alcoholic in early recovery is likely to develop a liking for sugar- and caffeine-loaded fizzy drinks, or more commonly diet versions, a pattern which I strongly challenge every time I see it. Keeping the appetite for sugar open in the alcoholic keeps a relapse in the wings, I believe.

In relation to eating disorders, many would suggest abstinence from sugar and white flour – and I agree that can work well, but it can also create the kind of unhelpful obsession that enables the focus to remain on the food (while neglecting the person). I think it important that whoever is suffering from an eating disorder decide where the boundary lies, which should be confirmed by their health professional, so that whatever they put in place to address the eating disorder comes from them and is therefore more likely to be maintained by them.

a. Anorexia

This is about restricting nourishment, not eating to the point of starvation, refusing food, becoming obsessive about food, how it's laid on a plate (e.g. the food groups mustn't touch each other), being very controlled and fussy around food, not being able to tolerate eating with people if eating at all, recoiling at the sound of chewing and denying any experience of hunger or appetite. Over and again, I meet families who cannot understand why their child won't eat even one grape and who battle to tempt their child to eat something.

There are two key dimensions that must be addressed with the anorexic, or, indeed, any eating disorder. The first is to establish an increasingly healthy eating pattern, where the right amount of calories or nourishment is taken in on a daily basis so that the weight can increase to a safe level and the brain return to 'normal functioning'. The second is to look at the psychopathology of anorexia which is 'to find safety in not needing'. Think about that. If the child has decided that their safety lies in not needing, then to admit an appetite, even for a grape, means their entire defence mechanism is broken down.

Anorexia will often attract overt caretaking, micromanagement of need and a desire to rescue in all those around the anorexic. On the surface, there is nothing more normal than wanting to go in and rescue someone as they become emaciated, but counter-intuitively this kind of micromanagement is exactly the kind of behaviour that enables the anorexic to stay locked down in not needing as others are prepared to step in and do things for them. The anorexic seeks to take up no space, no time, no food or resources, almost wiping themselves out from existing. This is an enormously angry action and may be felt as such by those around the anorexic. Recovery involves encouraging the anorexic to take up space, time, food and resources by talking and wanting and needing and making noise, all of which is tremendously difficult for them to do, but vital to counterbalance the sickness. To work out why your child has reverted to such extreme measures and to achieve a sense of safety are the first steps in knowing where to focus for yourself in your own recovery journey as the parent.

Early clues in your child may include not being hungry at mealtimes, pushing food around the plate, avoiding carbs, skipping breakfast or any meal, eating fruit and drinking lots of water (water-loading), an unhealthy focus on weight or a distorted view of their own weight. Often when someone is anorexic and they have a 'negative' emotion they will translate it through their weight and express feeling 'fat' instead of what they're really feeling. This is a red herring and the key is to remain with the feeling rather than try to adjust or challenge your child's perception of their own weight.

b. Bulimia

This is about wanting and needing, but not being able to receive and experience feeling nourished. Having an appetite, but not being able to digest. Most people who suffer from bulimia describe the condition as bingeing and purging, often with intermittent patterns of restricting. Hidden in plain view, the bulimic can maintain a fairly steady weight, all the while engaging in violent patterns of self-abuse, relating to overeating to the point of pain, followed by purging through making themselves sick, by the use of laxatives, through overexercise and sometimes through self-harm. I see bulimia as an act of rage and always include intensive anger work in a care plan.

The bulimic will eat and then feel discomfort or disgust to the point where they are compelled to get rid of whatever they have taken in the form of sustenance. This is about their right to receive nourishment and to benefit from the food. The bulimic often comes from a family where personal needs are not clear, or where a parent might deny their own need, so the child takes without knowing what is rightfully theirs. This can leave a child feeling rageful at the mixed messages, and shame for their appetite. Thus working with someone who is bulimic requires patience and time. They will need to eat little and often, in order to avoid feeling overfull (as this will trigger a compulsion to purge), all the while connecting with the buried emotions.

Interestingly, I have noticed that people who suffer from bulimia are also often almost bulimic in the way they talk and interact, as if purging their energy, and talking in volume and at a pace. Generally they also have difficulty receiving a compliment, whereas a criticism will almost always go all the way in.

Clues include drinking lots of liquids before eating as it makes vomiting easier, and then leaving the table mid-meal or immediately afterwards to go to the loo. Often a bulimic will run the shower or the tap to cover up for the sound of vomiting. You will see them display what many parents call a healthy appetite, although there is often a sweet tooth present and almost always a self-consciousness that means they will never really accept a compliment.

c. Overeating

Often known as comfort eating, people who are overeaters, or binge eaters, will eat and eat until they are in physical pain, unable to move or, and this is key, think about anything other than the pain. People feel profound shame as they believe that their pattern of overeating is greed, and they report levels of self-disgust and self-loathing that will prevent them from ever asking for help. Someone who is an overeater can overeat for years before it manifests as overweight or obesity. Sometimes an overeater will develop other forms of an eating disorder to try and compensate for the weight that they gain in their comfort eating. It can start by feeling increasingly hungry and having bigger portions which, of course, can go under the radar when kids are growing up as the disproportionate amount of food is put down to a healthy appetite, or even to a child being particularly active. If that child then also eats snacks in-between meals, it is worth considering whether the 'hunger' they are describing is a physical hunger that warrants more food or if it is an emotion that has been converted into a physical feeling so that there is something tangible to displace onto.

Every overeater I have ever known and worked with has expressed profound feelings of shame, loneliness and insecurity, and these feelings often form the basis of all the therapeutic work once the healthier eating pattern is in place. Interestingly, my experience of young people who are overeaters is that what they have in common is a desire to please their parent. It seems that they are taking from the parent something (i.e. food) that the parent is able to give, as if to prove to the parent that they (the parent) is good enough.

At the heart of an overheating problem is the inability to know what is enough, to experience satisfaction. Thus, at the very core of a successful treatment plan is teaching about what is enough in whatever form that might take; it is vital to re-educate the appetite.

It is worth noting that once somebody is clinically obese, the brain starts to change to accommodate that level of appetite, so bariatric surgery (weight-loss surgery that is only advised if a child is over fourteen years old and extremely overweight) alone is unlikely to deliver a sustainable solution without psychological or therapeutic intervention targeting how the brain acclimatises to the appetite. In other words, if you take extreme measures to reduce weight or to control your food intake don't expect your craving to stop unless you directly address it through medication (from a psychiatrist specialised in this area), alongside therapy.

Early clues of this condition include: an increasing appetite, second and third helpings, snacking, eating to fill a void, night eating, secret eating and finishing off other people's food, as well as a dismissal of need despite an unregulated appetite.

4. Sex and love addiction (also known as an intimacy and attachment disorder)

Always running hand in hand with dysregulated food patterns and a dysfunctional relationship with money, a person's experience of intimacy and relationship is a direct reflection of their relationship with themselves. I often look at sex and love addiction through the same lens as I do eating disorders in that I consider the person's experience of relationship as anorexic (I don't need), bulimic (I need, but I can't keep) or overeating (I don't know what is enough).

Hiding in 'not needing' might allow a child or teenager to feel safe if they can convince themselves they don't want to connect, but usually this comes from a core belief that 'if I do connect with you, you will reject or hurt me'. We are social creatures and although many people report feeling they need time on their own to recalibrate, we also need connection. In a bulimic-style relationship, there is always intensity-seeking behaviour and high drama so that one day the person is intensely close to someone, the next they have fallen out with them. And it's extreme: all or nothing/ binge and purge.

The relational 'overeater' will go one of two ways: they will either be promiscuous, and that can be sexual in whichever form it takes, or they will be anything to anyone in a relationship, just to be needed. This includes the needy person who will position themselves on the outskirts of, for example, the popular set and allow themselves to be exploited, to be the subject of jokes in order to establish a sense of belonging. They will put up with teasing and abuse, not knowing what is enough until they feel shame and withdraw into isolation. At school one way of spotting this is to note the pattern of the child who after every lesson needs a bit more time, who after every interaction needs just a bit more attention.

Working out relationships is an important part of the teenage experience and, indeed, that of any child. It is a core social motive that we belong, that we find our tribe. Social Influence Theory describes how we reinforce that sense of belonging not through affirming ourselves, but rather by criticising the other. To be confident in your sense of belonging in a group you are more likely to point and scorn those who you decide are different, rather than comment on what you all in your own group have in common. Of course, this creates feelings of power in the in-group and creates wishful thinking in those who don't belong – and it can be incredibly difficult for someone to navigate the social minefield.

5. Money

This goes hand in hand with the intimacy and attachment disorder and eating disorders. So far in my career, I have never met one without the others. A person's relationship with money is profoundly indicative of their relationship with themselves. There are fellowships like AA dedicated to underearners or debtors-people, who struggle to charge the right money for whatever it is that they do so that they offer their services for free or for less than market value. Learning how to both save and spend, give and receive in a healthy fashion, are fundamental requirements to living in a healthy way in Western society. Respecting that money has value, and knowing how to manage it as the currency by which we purchase items and services in our lives puts us in the driving seat. Someone who has an addiction around money will be driven by their fear of it: either having it or not having it, their shame around having or not having money and their sense of worth.

. . . .

> *I once worked with a family where the two teenagers had been brought up in a family of profound financial insecurity and each child had found a different way to 'control' their fear-based relationship with money. One was ambitious, placing money and the acquisition of money as a high priority so that he would never be without again, in perfect contrast to the other child, who appeared to be embarking upon a hippy-type existence, whereby money didn't matter at all.*

Money does matter: it is not everything, but it is the currency by which we live in our society and, as such, deserves respect. Relationships with money can follow the same patterns of that of an eating disorder or an attachment and intimacy disorder whereby it can be anorexic – I don't need; bulimic – I need but I spend easily; or an overeating pattern – I need and I don't know what is enough.

6. Gambling

Strange though it may seem, gambling is not necessarily about winning or losing, but it's about the playing. It is often about risk-taking, seeking to control or beat the system; it's about power. In my view, the original power is your same gender parent or caretaker and I see gambling as a representation of that power struggle as the gambler seeks to take on 'the machine', the machine that will always ultimately win. It is thus vital when treating a gambler, whether that's in rehab at the end of a long line of painful losses or as an early intervention, therapeutic work should be done with or relating to the same gender parent, because there inevitably will be a dimension of competition that has fuelled the self-destructive process.

Gambling is on the up as online access opens up the floodgates to middle-class and female gamblers. No longer relegated to the male-dominated corner bookies, seedy backroom or darkened casino, now gambling is readily available at your kitchen table, glass of Chablis in hand. You can gamble virtual money as the children sleep soundly in their IKEA beds, all the while stacking up real debt that will disturb their sense of financial security for ever. I am seeing more gamblers who are teenagers or young adults too, getting heavily into debt with loan companies, increasingly paranoid about opening emails or reading texts that chase payment as their debt relentlessly increases with the interest and they have no way to pay it, having already gambled their student loans. It's a desperate situation and one that forces young people into isolation, fear and crime to source quick money.

Gambling, as I say, is not always about winning money nor are the costs always financial. Gambling is as much about fighting the machine – the narcissistic hit of supremacy; it's about being driven to win back what you have lost already, in a financial sense but also, less consciously, in terms of identity and kudos. And even then, when you hit a winning streak, like a mosquito that plunges into an artery, you cannot pull out even though you know it's deadly. The compulsion, the denial, the cravings are all gambling's greatest henchman, shepherding you ever back into the fray to be beaten. The odds are not in your favour.

In my practice, I have worked with professional gamblers, some are parents like you and me, some are teenagers, and some are professionals from the corporate world – a number do financially very well. But the wake-up call is to notice at what cost, as inevitably their families suffer from their lack of emotional availability, the ever-changing financial status that can pitch between wealth and poverty, sometimes seemingly overnight, coupled with an often irritated and anxious state. I meet mothers ashamed, often under the guise of depression, as they seek help for the habit that has taken such hold that they have debts they cannot pay. I meet men who haven't told their wife yet that they are in over their heads. The easy access to gambling and apparently low stake offered makes for an innocuous-looking game at first look, but as the age-old joke goes: how do you make a small fortune? Start with a large one. You won't see the crash coming.

I have worked with young people living in terror, in debt to friends and to less friendly sources, unable to see a way out, at a place where suicide can seem like a good idea as they decline into hopelessness and despair. If you notice debts starting to rack up, ask your child why? Simply paying them off might only clear the way for more debt, so be proactive and ask questions.

7. Work

When a person's identity is bound up with what they do professionally and their self-esteem is gathered from their work experience, rather than having an inherent sense of self-worth, how they feel about themselves is constantly measured against their success (or failure) at work. Work addiction can be tricky to spot as it is socially reinforced as being 'hard-working/conscientious/diligent/ambitious'.

Often people find themselves working all the time, going into work earlier, not taking breaks, working late and then taking work home with them, wearing their work's demands almost as a badge of pride. Their conversation will be dominated by work; they will struggle to talk about anything else as it increasingly becomes their identity – and the office will love them, so any family concerns can be dismissed as jealousy or an attempt to control.

I have met successful business people who, on retirement, seem to suddenly develop alcohol dependence. Bewildered, they consult me to find out what's going on. In these situations, it becomes apparent that their pattern of working was so 'all or nothing' that when they stopped working it left a vacuum that demanded to be filled.

In children and teenagers, work addiction can manifest itself as perfectionism, overworking, hiding in schoolwork to avoid social activity and interaction, and it is often dismissed as relatively unimportant or a better alternative to drugs. I have even heard some parents say that they wish their child had this condition. But the hidden cost of this pattern of behaviour, which is so often encouraged and affirmed by parents and teachers alike when the child achieves great successes, is a fear of not being good enough. This self-doubt, this fear, will fuel a perfectionism that can end up almost paralysing that person from the ability to try. It can create anxiousness around exam times as they never know how much work is enough to maintain the grades that people have begun to expect of them. As this process continues, the child or teenager can start to feel increasingly isolated, as if their performance at school is everything they are. I can't count how many times I have been told by a teenager when I visit a school that they are really worried about what their parents will think if they don't do as well as they believe they should in their exams, expressing the fear of letting their parents down.

8. Exercise

Most parents want their child to take exercise for their best interests in terms of both physical and mental health, and the dangers of a sedentary lifestyle is ever more evident at the very least in the increasing obesity in our youth. But again, as with any other addiction, it is how that exercise is used that is key. How, why and how much is what we are looking to consider. For example, when somebody uses exercise to avoid or purge how they feel, they are engaging in what I would consider to be an addictive process, the negative consequences of which would include abandonment of self. If a person feels angry and goes for a run to burn off or get rid of that anger so that when they come back they don't feel that emotion then I would suggest they are simply setting themselves up for a dependence on exercise as a way of coping every time they feel angry. If, on the other hand, the person uses exercise as a way of managing their feelings so that they better understand themselves and when they have returned from a run, for example, they are able to better represent what has been going on for them and why they are angry, then there is no problem.

Many people with eating disorders will use exercise as a way to control the impact food has on their weight or body shape, so that they literally plan what physical activity they will do as they eat something to compensate for the weight they believe they would otherwise put on. Some people with eating disorders will literally jog on the spot to burn calories, insist on walking instead of taking a bus or taking the stairs instead of the lift.

An exercise addict is likely to do exercise to the point of self-harm so that they may experience physical damage as a result of the overt exercise regime which they will seek to cover up. They will be consumed by their interest in exercise, whether that be a sport, running, cycling, and will often seek validation about how well they look as a result. They will be distracted from everyday life, relationships, work, emotions, so that the exercise becomes the most important event in the week, about which everything else is positioned. Perhaps it is surprising to understand that what may have started out as making somebody feel good from the increased endorphins as a result of the exercise may become something that motivates self-loathing.

9. Nicotine

One of the most addictive substances is nicotine and it is also the most readily available and widely accepted habit despite recent changes to legislation. Teenagers continue to smoke as an assertion of independence and rebellion, alongside other reasons like appetite suppression and out of anxiousness. Smoking is an easy and accessible way of looking like an adult but, as we know, with potential long-term health consequences.

Dependence on nicotine often forms when a cigarette is used to do an emotional job. For example, smoking when you're bored means you never learn how to deal with being bored; smoking to take a break is a common use of cigarettes and without the cigarette I have witnessed a person's difficulty to stop for a moment; using a cigarette to cope when you are angry means you never learn how to handle your anger; having a cigarette to connect to people means you never learn how to simply make that connection without that prop, and so on and so on.

10. Caffeine

Here I am referring to the various caffeine-loaded drinks that are used as mixers or in health drinks to give you an energy boost, rather than to tea or coffee although, of course, they play their part. Readily available in shops, newsagents and garages, caffeine- and sugar-loaded drinks (which appeal to those with disordered eating patterns too) are commonly used by alcoholics as mixers, as mood lifters and as energy stimulants, with caffeine assuming its place as a staple in most people's diets in Western culture. Profoundly affecting mood, appetite, sleep patterns and, therefore, overall well-being, caffeine is an everyday drug that warrants closer attention, especially when somebody complains of sleep, mood or appetite disturbance, or is suffering from depressive or anxious symptoms.

It is not uncommon for teenagers as they approach their exams to also take caffeine pills as stimulants, in the belief that they will enhance their ability to stay awake and study successfully. The common downside is a crash in mood that can result in a profound state of anxiousness or depression, which, in turn, may end up being medicated as no one asks questions about the level of caffeine intake.

11. Screens

Smartphones, game consoles and laptop screens have begun to dominate our children's worlds and we are none of us sure what the long-term effects will be. What we do know is that they operate on the same neural pathways as drugs and alcohol, for example, so it is ever more critical that we teach our children how to manage their use of screens, their ability to pick up and put them down and to challenge dissociation and escape through using a screen in order to prevent a seamless transition into alcohol or drug addiction later in life. Children as young as two are commonly given a tablet, laptop or phone to keep them amused, to soothe or placate or just to keep them quiet. Whichever it is, in a way this inadvertently teaches them how to disconnect from their feelings and their behaviours – whereas the initial goal was perhaps to give the parent peace. What is being taught here instead are the first crucial steps in dissociating, in avoiding perfectly natural and normal feelings and behaviours at what are key stages of development. I believe we will witness, as a result, the knock-on effect of these children growing up without the skills necessary to handle their emotions and subsequent behaviours.

Many children spend in excess of eight hours a day on a screen on a regular basis, as their main form of leisure and communication with their peers. Many of these games have their design informed by psychology so that they are deliberately addictive, continually drawing the child to stay on for longer and making ending extremely difficult. Many of the games are also stimulating and aggressive, causing the child to be hypervigilant to attack, thereby generating adrenaline. No wonder then that when that game is interrupted for example by a parent exasperated by the length of time the child has been on, that they are met with an explosive tantrum that can only apparently be calmed by the return of the device.

I'm often asked if screens are actually addictive and my answer is 'yes', on the premise that they are used to self-medicate and to detrimental effect that commonly includes dependence, volatile mood, neediness as in the case of extreme dependence on social media likes and validation of self through others' eyes, isolation, disturbed appetite and sleep pattern, negative impact on learning and social anxiety. Unfortunately, screen use is not always considered as part of a mood disorder assessment. So if your child is suffering mental health symptoms, it's vital you mention their screen use to your GP or consultant.

But technology is not going away and it is vital that we learn how we use screens so that we are using them for our advantage and pleasure rather than becoming a slave to our device. Learning how to intervene on an evolving screen addiction is possible, even in the most extreme cases, but it requires you, the parent, to resist the provocations that your child will inevitably throw at you when you intervene, and learning to teach what other things your child could do instead. This is nowhere near as easy as it sounds in a world where technology dominates, and being proactive can feel like inviting trouble. Have faith, as if you intervene in a clear and respectful way, are consistent in your approach and hold the boundary, change can happen. It's easier the younger the child is, so start as soon as you can and resist the temptation to use screens as a babysitter.

12. Self-harm

In its simplest form this is an attempt to release emotion through physical injury such as cutting, burning, pinching, scratching, hitting, banging head against a hard surface, pulling eyebrows/lashes out, pulling hair out, or even inviting being hit. I would add talking to yourself abusively as self-harming behaviour, as the effect is to purge negative emotion, while causing negative impact on self. People who self-harm often develop an intimate relationship with their particular process, and the resulting scars, so that they will experience almost a pride around how they damage themselves alongside a sense of shame, as they usually know that what they're doing is not right, and crucially also envy if they see somebody else's scars.

13. Codependence

This is what I call the socially acceptable face of addiction, posing as love, care, loyalty and friendship yet driven by low self-worth and pain. It is such an important form of addiction that it is also covered in more detail in Chapter 5. Codependence is 'conditional giving presented as unconditional giving'. As a codependent, you are likely to say 'don't worry about me, let's worry about you' and feel (but rarely say) 'after all I've done for you, and you treat me like this . . .'. Codependency represents the hurt and overlooked experience of the person who gives in order to achieve belonging, status and identity, and who gives more than they can afford in terms of time, energy, attention and other physical resources such as money. On the receiving end, you are likely to feel trapped or obliged but not know why. You may feel as if you are a bad person for wanting to hurt or reject the codependent giver.

Wherever there is an addict or someone high maintenance, there will be the wing man, the emotional shock absorber, and that is the codependent, primed to overlook their own needs in favour of the overt need or demand of the other.

14. Shopping (and shoplifting)

So much more than 'retail therapy', shopping as an addictive process will lead someone to be driven to seek out items, e.g. clothing, cosmetics, technology, jewellery, household items, cars, whatever they believe will redefine them as somebody of worth. Buying identity through an external item will take the shopaholic through a roller coaster of feelings that starts with planning, anticipation, choosing and buying, after which comes the steep decline of shame, fear and what many describe as feeling hollow. Much of the time, the shopaholic is too embarrassed to return the items they have bought, so they remain in their original packaging hidden away in their cupboards like skeletons waiting to be discovered. Of course, the consequences will be financial, but the critical consequence is the shame a person feels when they realise that they have once again engaged in this self-defeating circuit, and the loss of time. With so much opportunity on sites like eBay, Amazon and Depop and many others like them, it is all too easy for teens to overspend from the privacy of their bedrooms as part of a desperate bid to belong.

Shoplifting too can be 'addictive'. The adrenaline rush planning to steal something, anything, just to beat 'the machine' or take on authority, can be intoxicating. I have noticed over the years that shoplifting often goes hand in hand with other addictive behaviours – bulimia and gambling – with a competitive edge, taking without permission, often getting something you don't even want, perhaps not even wanting to acknowledge your own need, being common themes.

15. Obsessive Compulsive Disorder (OCD)

Extreme forms of OCD may not be treated successfully through an addiction model alone, however, some of the principles that underlie OCD form part of the thinking behind this approach to addiction and which it seeks to address. If you consider the basic premise of OCD as an attempt to control the person's external world (which is impossible) in order to achieve some sense of internal calm, safety or peace – which will inevitably generate anxiousness – it falls in line with this model of addiction. OCD can come in many forms, such as counting patterns, organising items in the environment, walking patterns, checking patterns, behavioural patterns, cleaning patterns, all of which are designed to control and thereby create a sense of safety. The desire to control, the need to control to irrational lengths is usually driven by a profound sense of feeling unsafe. It is a core social motive (Fiske, 2009) to have a sense of control in one's life. However as with other addictive processes, OCD can quickly take over a person's life to the exclusion of everything else. So if you notice that your child wants things, needs things done or presented in a particular way, whether that's related to their clothes, their bedroom, their food, timings, washing, etc. – whatever it is that becomes their focus, it forms an increasingly non-negotiable routine or pattern – then I would suggest that you start to consider what might be driving this need for control rather than focus on trying to reason them out of whatever it is they are imposing upon you and your family. Trying to challenge the OCD pattern is likely to generate frustration and irritation and therefore anxiousness in the child, who will then need to compensate through further OCD behaviours. The need for safety must be addressed as a priority so that the child does not find sanctuary in a particular pattern, regime or in their perfectionism (which will probably go on to cause procrastination).

Questions:
- Do you use any of these manifestations to help cope with how you feel or with what's going on in your life?
- Do they help? Or are they causing problems, hidden or overt? (Be specific.)
- What do you think you are teaching your child as a result?
- What behaviour or patterns of 'using' are you worried about in your child?
- Given what you may have read, why do you think your child is 'using'?

These fifteen manifestations describe how addiction shows up in someone, in your teenager, in your child, with each relapse making the addiction stronger, the family more distant and recovery feel less possible. But the key is this. Addiction can dominate family and relationship experience before showing up as a recognisable manifestation and it is here that we must focus to achieve early intervention. This is the 'root system' or The Core Characteristics™ of addiction.

4

THE CORE CHARACTERISTICS™

No one airdrops into chronic addiction, so what comes before?

Addiction operates on a continuum and to effectively intervene before it manifests as chronic, it's important to start further back down that continuum, noticing what drives the using behaviours, the emotions and thoughts and intervening constructively. If you want to parent in a way that proactively seeks to prevent addiction as outlined in the last chapter, you have to know where to focus.

The Core Characteristics™ is a list of human characteristics which I have collated as a result of decades of experience and which I believe are pivotal in the prevention of addiction. In my view, to overlook them is to miss a vital opportunity of early intervention and prevention of addiction, as this is where the action is not only to get into recovery (as opposed to constantly firefighting just to remain clean and sober), but also to prevent addiction through the promotion of emotional intelligence, resilience and self-esteem.

It is not a new concept in psychology to try and encapsulate the motivational needs and wants of the successful evolution of human beings in society. In 2007, psychologist Susan Fiske conceptualised five core social motives, a popular needs model forming the acronym BUC(k)ET which stands for: Belonging, Understanding, Controlling, Enhancing self and Trusting. In this model, Belonging is the essential core social motive, which the others all service or facilitate to enable effective functioning in social groups. It assumes the motivation to bond as a way to create connection, the requirement to feel competitive and effective, a need to feel appreciated or socially worthy and acknowledges that your perspective of the world affects your sense of peace or increased suspicion and vigilance.

Abraham Maslow conceptualised the eight basic needs (Maslow, 1943) which he introduced as: physiological (basic self-care facilitates balanced mood), safety, belonging, self-esteem, cognitive (to learn, explore, discover and create), aesthetic, self-actualisation (striving) and self-transcendence (spiritual).

Similarly, The Core Characteristics™ of addiction are normal, ordinary human characteristics that everyone can identify with, but that for people like me, and for some of your children, are experienced in such extreme ways that they are the breeding ground for the aggressive self-destructive pattern that is addiction. If you are proactive in how you parent, you can begin to address these as part of your child's growing up process, irrespective of whether they display a problem or not. Most addiction treatment programmes recognise a need for a reparenting approach, teaching the addict to learn to parent themselves more kindly and apply better self-care. Taking its guide from this approach, this model aims to help you, the parent, to be the parent you want to be in the first place so the vacuum for a reparenting process is avoided.

It can be difficult to identify whether your child is using something in a harmful way or not, and you have a choice as to whether you stand by and watch, fingers crossed, hoping they grow out of it, or if you intervene. Using The Core Characteristics™ as a guide allows you to intervene through being a proactive parent in a way that won't cause harm; you have nothing to lose and everything to gain.

The list is as follows. If they are noticed and respected as aspects of a person's development requiring attention, guidance and compassion, I firmly believe this can provide the basis for prevention of developing addiction.

1. Control

When people refer to 'control' they are often describing their experience of somebody else as being very controlling, or 'a control freak', a term that is shaming and absolute. As a result, control or the need to control is usually perceived as a bad thing and something to avoid admitting. Somebody being controlling, or being perceived as controlling, also allows those around them to relinquish responsibility in the face of the power that controlling person apparently has. So the observation of somebody being controlling has with it an association of blame. Yet as we can see from many psychological views, having a sense of control or agency over your environment or circumstance is fundamental to an experience of well-being. Thus conflict around this basic human need is the most significant in determining the likelihood of addiction to develop.

Control and vulnerability

Control is how we manage our vulnerability, and I view addiction as a behavioural pattern of avoiding being vulnerable at any cost. Although this is an unconscious mission statement – 'I will not be vulnerable (again)' – the behaviour is to manipulate the impact of everything that affects that person's world even if it causes worse trouble or pain. This might be because the individual has experienced some sort of trauma where they have felt hurt or afraid as a result of not being in control, it may be due to a particular sensitivity in the child or in the family culture that heightens vigilance (and therefore fear). Whatever it is that has caused this defensive pattern, it can quickly take on a life of its own. Someone suffering in this way will not be able to bear not knowing what people think of them, so will instead take control and create life on their terms, perhaps through people-pleasing or provocation that can feel difficult for others to understand.

. . . .

Jenny was a girl in her teens who believed she was difficult to get on with, and had come to see me because she felt angry all the time and most of her relationships – both in how she behaved and how she was treated – were aggressive. There was always a drama and the presence of threatened or actual violence. She talked about her childhood and her experience of a father who had singled her out in the family as the only one he ever hit. Jenny felt it was something about her that had warranted the violence; although it had not been frequent, it had often come out of nowhere as far she was concerned. Through letting her guard down and trusting the therapeutic environment (becoming vulnerable), Jenny was able to connect with her fear and hurt as a child. Although her father's violence was inexcusable, she realised that she had provoked him, not out of defiance as she had previously thought, nor because she was 'difficult', but because she had needed to control what she had learned was inevitable. The only thing she could control was the timing of the violence, so she did. Jenny had inevitably gone on to apply this provocative identity in all her subsequent relationships, inadvertently confirming herself as the common denominator in her aggressive interaction, as the problem. The therapy helped her to hold her father to account, in her mind's eye, and to accept her resulting profound fear of vulnerability which had led her to behave in a way that was initially to protect herself, but which had gone on to cause her a great deal of unhappiness. Forgiving herself, she could begin to react differently and be kinder to herself when she felt afraid.

I have met adults and teenagers who have learned to people-please in order to feel safe, trying to control what other people think of them, which is usually driven by fear. Much of the time the adult has forgotten the originating fear, and described instead a constant sense of anxiety around interactions with others. Reacting through compliance or defiance, the child doesn't actually learn and grow, they just do as they're told while rebelling in their head (a time bomb waiting to go off) or they openly defy. Too often time-poor parents will demand compliance because of their own time constraints, stress or need to control. But just as frequently that parent will be met with defiance and it is here that a very real challenge begins for the parent to be curious rather than offended, to step away from the ego that might retaliate with the reaction 'how dare you speak to me like that', and to **reconsider exactly that question instead: how do they dare? And what do they need?** In teaching a healthy relationship between control and vulnerability, parents give the child vital steps towards independence and healthy interdependence. Crucially, an unhealthy relationship in this area will demand self-medication, to repress the real feelings as they have had no place in the home.

Questions:
- List five ways you seek to control how you feel.
- Why?
- List five ways you seek to control another's behaviour.
- Why?
- List five ways you think your child is controlling you/the family (or trying to).
- Why might this be?
- Is your behaviour helpful and respectful or are you fuelling something negative with how you are responding?
- What have you learned?

2. Denial

Denial is the process of taking any given bit of information, altering it in some way, and then talking or acting from there. This means that the person is less vulnerable as there is a filter between what actually happened and the reconstructed version. To be a bit more specific, denial can take several forms: generalising – it happens all the time; universalising – everybody does it; minimising – it was only once/wasn't that bad; exaggerating – it was the worst thing ever; justifying – it was because you shouted at me. Through a process of denial, the experience is vitally changed and turned into something else. This means that in any subsequent discussion, actions taken or assurances made are relevant to a distortion of the truth.

There are so many examples I could give of the denial that I have witnessed and experienced for myself with varying degrees of importance, but all are fundamentally the same. There is the proud young man who came to me because his parents were worried about his levels of anxiousness. He would come in on a pushbike and one day I noticed his trousers were torn at the knee. I asked him what had happened and he told me it was nothing. Gently insisting, I asked him to explain what had actually happened and he reluctantly told me that he had come off his bike as he tried to cycle onto the pavement off the road. This had made him feel stupid and self-conscious so that his first reaction had been to look around to see who had seen this happen rather than to check he was OK. He had dismissed his hurt knee instead feeling shame for falling off. Crucially it was he who was judging himself, thinking himself stupid, convinced others would agree. This incident was on a micro-level compared to other forms of denial but I bring it because he had suffered for many years from anxiety and it was in this detail that we started to gain access to his angry relationship with himself and resulting poor self-esteem.

In more extreme examples, I have met many parents who have ignored their gut instinct as a child returns drunk from a social gathering more and more frequently. They explain it away as one-off circumstance each time, or one parent persuades the other to just let it go, believing their child will grow out of it. When the pungent smell of weed starts hanging heavily around their teen, it can scare parents, who prefer to ignore it and hope it goes away – if they acknowledge it they feel obliged to do something and often they don't know what that should be. Sometimes, of course, parents don't think weed is an issue, they might even smoke it 'occasionally' themselves. But if as you watch your teenager struggling you feel so deskilled and out of touch with them, if you ask yourself how on earth you got here, my guess would be that part of the journey was by denial. For whatever reason the clues were ignored or were left unchallenged, so no pattern was ever established that might have raised the flag sooner. But if you do intervene early enough, even then denial can get in the way as you perceive the suggestion from a therapist too extreme and so refuse the therapy they offer, saying you'll come back it if gets worse. Why wait? Decent therapy won't do any harm! Running a Family Support Group every week, I meet parents with children who are in a critical condition, sitting opposite parents who are worried by formative signs of trouble. The latter often feel fraudulent as their problems seem so much less than everyone else's, the former are regretful that they hadn't accessed help sooner. It's hard to take your own problems seriously – neither exaggerating nor minimising, just seeing them for what they are and responding appropriately.

Questions:
- In the last week have I used any of the following denial patterns to avoid being vulnerable and honest with someone?
  - Exaggeration (making something more than it was to emphasise my point).
  - Minimising (making something less than it was to try and avoid dealing with it).
  - Universalising (making something seem normal because everyone does it).
  - Justifying (making it inevitable that I did or said something because of something or someone else).
- Did I feel powerful (self-righteous and angry) or powerless (ashamed and worthless) as a result?
- Where are those feelings now? How did I deal with them?
- What have I learned?

3. Deceit, secrets and lies

A pattern of not telling the truth is *always* present in any addictive process because that dishonesty allows that person to create a false reality that prevents them from feeling vulnerable. It's a way of staying separate from yourself. Common patterns also include not admitting fault, having a superior attitude, not being clear, warping reality, picking holes in others. No one who suffers from addiction trusts anyone, choosing instead to trust their 'drug of choice' as their closest confidant. When you don't trust, you lie. 'I'm fine' (when I'm dying inside), 'no thanks, I don't need any help/comfort/friendship'(when I feel crippled by my isolation), 'it wasn't me' (when it was but I can't face it), 'it's not that bad' (when I'm terrified it was the worst), 'lots of my friends smoke weed, but I don't. I tried it but it makes me feel sick' (when actually I'm the biggest stoner in the group), 'I've already eaten' (when I haven't eaten all day), 'I don't need any money thanks, I'm using my savings' (when I've stolen from your purse, or sold drugs to friends to make some cash). Mostly an addict will believe their own lies, which is the real reason they are often so convincing.

Surrounded by secrets and reconstructions of the truth the addict seeks to hide from being known, even from themselves. Sometimes the lies can be pointless so there doesn't appear to be any reason to lie, just so that others don't actually know what they're doing. It doesn't mean they're doing anything wrong; they just don't want to be honest (or to be known and seen).

Others might tell elaborate lies, weaving an intricate web of an alternate version of themselves or their life, even enjoying the deception as a form of control. But this ultimately backfires through isolating them from genuine connection with others.

It's worth noting too that secrets in a family set up a culture of deceit, and those secrets may be because something is covered up. Children will often sense this discrepancy and react to it without even realising, becoming manipulative and duplicitous as a way of getting their needs met indirectly.

Questions:
- Does my child lie to me?
- About what?
- How do I respond?
- Is my response designed to manipulate my child to open up to me or am I genuinely curious?
- Am I honest or do I have secrets?

- Do I have self-respect and do I treat myself with self-respect?
- Why should my child trust me? Am I trustworthy or do I get over-involved, overreact or put him or her down?
- Why do I want an honest relationship with my child?

4. Fear

There are two well-known acronyms for FEAR in the world of addiction that say it all – F*** Everything And Run – or Face Everything And Recover.

Addiction is driven by fear: the fear of other people's opinions or reaction or abandonment, loneliness, criticism or abuse, being exposed, trapped or not having control – of being vulnerable. These kinds of self-centred fears will isolate you from human connection.

Of course, many people who suffer from addiction have experienced in their childhoods things that made them very afraid. As a result, some dissociate entirely from fear, seeming fearless, and others become consumed by it. Without a balanced experience of this important quality, it is hard to assess danger and so many people in addiction find themselves in life-threatening situations without even really noticing. They often cannot see how they got there, or what they might have done different. Or they are paralysed by fear and more than risk averse, they are life averse. Either way the addict is also often plagued by the fear that they are a fraud, and will one day be found out. And in a way it's true, as they are so fearful of being vulnerable that the defence is to create a version of themselves that performs in the world and so in a way is fraudulent. Always on the run, the addict fears being caught, seen and connected – because if we connect my fear is that I am not who you think I am (and then you'll reject me). Successfully teaching a child to manage this important emotion so that it informs them, so they can make choices that are in their interest and so that they are not paralysed by their fear comes from the experience of overcoming fear, over and again, and from realising that 'this too will pass'.

The instinct of the parent to protect their child and take their pain and fear away needs the manual override of knowing that a child needs to face their consequences in order to grow up into a healthy, independent adult. If your child has unreasonable fears, whether that's in the form of nightmares, self-confidence or social anxiety, the more you rescue the more you endorse the need for rescue. It's important for a child to feel heard and supported, but also for the adult to assess the situation and give a calm guide so that the child can trust and realign themselves to a healthier way of thinking or behaving. If the parent is impatient or angry, or at the other end of the scale, fearful and rescuing, then the child will probably feel unable to receive any advice or reassurance. They are then left alone with their fears.

Questions for you and/or your child:
- What does fear feel like to you?
- Notice the urgency to respond (fight/flight/freeze).
- Where do you feel it in your body?
- How does your personality change when you feel afraid?
- Is this how you want to be?
- What/why do you fear for your child?
- How do you relate to this?
- What do you do when you feel fear that you might not do if you felt safe?
- What are you teaching through modelled behaviour around fear? For example, anxiety (another form of fear!).

Actions:
- Make five promises to yourself around how you will behave in future when you feel fear.
- Look at your hand, see its age and shape and recognise it as part of you in the right now. Place your hand over the part of your body that feels the fear (i.e. your chest or your stomach) and allow the warmth of your hand (today) reach and soothe the old fear that resides inside you from old unresolved experiences (the past). Allow yourself to parent yourself so that you can hear the fear, see if it has any real foundation and decide what action you do or don't need to take, but calmly and with self-respect.

5. Shame

There are two distinct forms of shame, one is healthy and one is toxic. We need the first, but the second is dangerous.

Healthy shame

This is the experience of embarrassment or even guilt when you overstep a known boundary that reflects your moral code. It could be described as a conscience or even as a reflection of somebody's mature relationship with society. It's when you know you've done something wrong, irrespective of your desire to justify what you've done, and handled properly, you learn from the experience.

As parents I believe it is part of our role to introduce this moral code to our children so that, as they grow up, they internalise similar values that allow them to be independently productive and respectful as part of society (society being the extension of family). This means that we teach them manners, that we teach them the difference between right and wrong, acceptable and unacceptable behaviour and the concept of respect. It means if they steal something, they feel guilty, even if they are not caught, because they have overstepped a moral boundary. If they hit or bite a friend in the playground, they need to feel embarrassed and guilty as a reflection of the healthy shame that will teach them that behaviour is not acceptable. These lessons and moral codes are taught most successfully through modelled behaviour and consistent, understandable boundaries.

Dangerous or toxic shame

Healthy shame becomes toxic shame when the child believes that it is them that is wrong as opposed to their behaviour. In other words, 'I am wrong', as opposed to 'I am **in the** wrong'. This subtle but vital difference is key in believing there is nothing I can do because there is something so deeply wrong with me that I have to hide, as opposed to there is something wrong with my behaviour that I need to change. If I believe there is something deeply wrong with me, I will anticipate the agony of rejection and abandonment in all that I do, and so I will never let you close. Further I will never let anything matter, and I will self-medicate against my vulnerability so that I don't feel it, even if what I use to alter my feelings causes me harm.

. . . .

I met Mia just after she turned sixteen years old. Her sense of esteem was so damaged that she provoked me to reject her from the moment we met. She was quite rude and critical of the reception-ist, the room, even my shoes, and was quite clear that she thought therapy was 'a load of bull'. I noticed how I felt in her company and wondered at the emotional response I was having, a vital clue that she was seeking to control what I thought of her. I realised her shame-based identity was driving what she felt was the inevitable – rejection – so she sought to make it happen and showed herself to be a waste of time. She was convincing too, and it took several ses-sions for her to realise that I remained curious rather than drawn into either fight her view or comply with it. It took several sessions for her also to begin to even notice me as a person (not a stranger or 'another therapist'). After that, we slowly began to build the trust that allowed us to explore her painful experiences of relationship.

It is impossible for someone to be in good self-esteem and/or experience intimacy if they are in toxic shame, thus it is of fundamental importance to proactively parent against this damaging characteristic. For a parent in terms of communicating good/bad, right/wrong, a simple adjustment to make is to focus on the behaviour rather than on the child themselves when either criticising or affirming. This means that the child is told that whatever they are doing is, for example, rude, obstructive, resistant, difficult to understand rather than that they are rude, obstructive, resistant, difficult to understand. In addition to this it is useful to remember that your view is a subjective view, and to include that when you speak. This then extends beyond telling the child that whatever it is they are doing is, for example, difficult to understand and adding yourself in relationship with that child so that what you actually say is 'I **find** your behaviour difficult to understand'.

Too often as parents, we point the finger at the child, forgetting it's our view and therefore subjective, loaded by our perceptions and expectations, which we are often in denial of anyway.

In addition, to notice that what we criticise in others is probably something we don't like about ourselves is a useful exercise in humility; this is called 'spot it you got it'.

Actions:
- Try to honestly consider if you shame your child.
- Consider why you might have done this – did it come from your own childhood experience, e.g. worrying about what others might think?
- Think about how you might change if you do.
- Try affirming your child more often for things that they have done – little things like clearing up or being kind or polite are just as important as bigger successes.
- Notice their reaction. Be sincere and don't overdo it: little and often is the way to create sustainable change.
- If your child resists accepting help or comfort from you, then try to respond with compassion. There will be a reason.
- When you want to criticise, give the message with compassion.
- If your child bristles or is defensive, it suggests they're taking it personally, perhaps because in the past you've meant it personally. Reinforce that it's the behaviour you're addressing, not them personally – no one is perfect!

6. Compulsion

Compulsion can be understood as a lack of impulse control, long since recognised as an implicit part of addiction. However more than just having the feeling that you have to do something no matter what, it's the very fact that it's the feelings that are driving the behaviour that is so significant about this particular characteristic. This means that whatever someone does or doesn't do is based on how they feel, or what they think they want or don't want, which means plans become unreliable. It also means people start to do what they want rather than what they need, which is a vital distinction to be aware of when bringing up children because they don't always want what they need.

Known as the f*** it button, commitments get changed or cancelled at the last minute, often based on a mood swing, and perceptions are all over the place. We all struggle with our feelings at times, but some people more than others, and if your emotions have too much power in decision-making, then they will begin to drive those decisions.

. . . .

I met Jacqui when she was thirty-four. An attractive woman, she was lonely but rarely went to social events for fear of feeling awkward and this had been going on since she left university. Sometimes having said 'yes' to an invitation, she would almost immediately start thinking about ways to get out of it. Desperate to meet someone and start a family, she could feel opportunity slipping away with every year. Her fear drove her decision to isolate and her self-esteem suffered as a result as her dream of becoming a mother became ever more distant. Alongside dismantling the events that had initiated this negative coping pattern, helping her to see that feelings are not facts and that although she needed to listen to them, her feelings didn't have to dictate her behaviour – compulsion – was groundbreaking for her.

It's important to encourage your child to follow through on any given plan, irrespective of how they feel, unless when it's a genuine emergency of some kind. Whether that's in relation to joining a club or taking up an instrument or going to a friend's house or agreeing to walk the dog on Wednesday. Whatever it is, it's important they follow it through and don't persuade you to allow them to change plans, even moving the commitment to the next day, just because they are tired or angry or caught up in a drama.

In rehab, we promote weekly plans so that people write down their week in advance – including what they plan to eat and when, and even when they have nothing to do – and follow it through. Throughout the day, there will be reasons to change the plan to accommodate life and things that come up that are more attractive or give an opportunity to opt out, but it is a fundamental part of the programme to have the feelings and be tempted to change, but to do what you said you would do all the same. This promotes learning to make commitments you can keep; being realistic, following through; reliability and self-discipline and being able to tolerate difficulty; resilience – and that's for starters. It also makes people think about the commitment they make.

Prevention is better than cure and if your child learns this discipline when they are young then the teen years should be a lot easier, for both of you!

Actions:
Try writing a plan for yourself – or help your child to write one – and put in everything you will do and at what time. See what it's like to stick to the plan, not deviating for anything other than a genuine emergency. The plan can be for a day, or even an hour to start with, but you need to slowly build confidence over two or three weeks to being able to plan a week at a time. Once this is in place, you will see a difference as the short-term predictability can help create stability and also make space for spontaneity.
- How did you/your child feel writing it?
- How did your child feel following it?
- When did your child want to deviate – why?
- What were they trying to gain or avoid?
- Why? What does this tell you about your child that you can help them with?

7. Obsession

As an addiction develops so do the levels of obsession, which can manifest in many ways but all have in common a single-minded intensity. People can get really stuck in patterns and routines and fixate on days of the week or times of the day as significant so that they can project all week, either looking forward to or looking back on that moment or experience, thereby being very busy-minded but never in the right now. This 'busy mind' is a form of obsession that means a person is consumed by worry or by a person or a thing – to the exclusion of anything else.

I have known people who have believed that they are in control of their drinking or drug taking because they only use it on a designated day every week and they present this evidence with pride as if it is evidence of their self-control and therefore their right to continue drinking or whatever it is. What quickly becomes clear though is that on the days that they are *not* using they are thinking about using, planning it or reliving it so that their obsession dominates their life. The same goes for those so obsessed by their work that they are not available for the relationships in their families, even getting intolerant when their loved ones complain about how little they see them. Yet that's a compliment! Or list-makers who obsessively note down all the things that they want to do and that they should do in an attempt to be organised or productive. Instead it backfires into an inflexible pattern of list-making that leaves everyone around them feeling micro-managed and suffocated, and the person themselves left frustrated and overwhelmed by how much they always have to do. Obsession takes you to a different world where you live separately from other people and any challenge to the obsession will simply drive it underground.

* *

Rose was so obsessed by an ex-boyfriend that every day when she got up she would dress in a way that she thought he would like, just in case she bumped into him. She lived in London. It's a big city with a low percentage of a chance meeting. The fantasy that ran through her mind, the various conversations she ran in her head just in case they should meet and the hypervigilance that expected him everywhere meant that she was lost in her obsession for him and oblivious to any current opportunity or experience, especially if it was another relationship. Rose felt so ashamed about how much she thought about him that she had stopped talking about him to her friends and had sought therapy as a forum to discuss the object of her obsession. Unfortunately (for her addiction), I believed this would only serve to feed the obsession, and so instead of talking about him, I worked to help her explore beneath the obsession to see what was driving her need to be so consumed with someone else.

Thinking is an important part of any process, but out of balance it can feel like having one foot on the accelerator and the other on the brake – watch the engine blow.

Actions:
Commit ninety seconds three times each day – breakfast, lunch and supper time – to find a private place to practise this discipline:
1. Set your phone alarm for ninety seconds.
2. Sit somewhere private. Both feet on the floor. Palms on tops of thighs. Eyes closed. Focus on the breath between nose and mouth, nothing else, that's all.

(I bet you struggle to go further than fifty-five seconds the first few times and check your phone in case you mis-set the alarm!)

8. Projection

This is a pattern of avoiding being in the present, in the here and now. It places someone in yesterday or tomorrow, fretting over what happened or could have been. This pattern of projection can really cement somebody into a negative core belief with no way out and can often be mistaken for anxiety.

Annabel found it difficult to concentrate in lessons; such was her perfectionism that all she focused on was what she thought she was missing. Thus at the end of every lesson she needed a conversation with the teacher and would ask several of her peers for what the homework was, for clarification. This would often elicit irritation in those around her, which left her feeling panicked. She would frequently attend the staffroom at the end of the day and ask for help from whichever teacher answered the door. But what was apparent was that no matter how much help she got it didn't make a difference to her anxious neediness. In only a few sessions, and then subsequently through a meeting with her teachers, she was able to alter this pattern. What was key was to bring her into the moment so that instead of thinking of what the final essay would look like, she learned to simply focus on reading a chapter and making one page of notes. At the core was a distrust of the advice she was getting as she was used to her mother reassuring her simply because she (her mother) could not tolerate Annabel's fear. Learning to trust the feedback from the teachers was life-changing for Annabel as it allowed her to simply follow direction. For her teachers, they had to commit to telling her to do the best she could with what she had when she came knocking on the staffroom door for help, and to give it in as planned. This stopped them feeling obliged to step in and fix, and it prevented Annabel from using her fear to control the teaching staff to give her answers and, in so doing, justify her low self-esteem. It also helped her to see the level of her ability as a fact.

The pattern of projection is a well-practised distraction away from whatever is happening in the moment, and it is a powerful way to dissociate while looking connected. There are feelings and thoughts and interactions, all of which look like a full and busy life, but what is key is the lack of connection in the moment.

It is important to note that in any pattern where somebody is hard on themselves, or prone to beating themselves up, there will be a great deal of projection as part of the process.

Actions:
Getting into the present from your own anxious projections when you are trying to support a child to do the same requires patience and calm parenting skills. The two important points are that: i) nothing can be done while bouncing around in your head; ii) bouncing around in your head makes you feel worse.

1. Acknowledge the facts.
2. Call it projection – a damaging avoidance tactic.
3. Breathe – in for five and out for seven counts.
4. Describe things in your immediate environment – the more specific, the more present you have to be.
5. Once present, write down the facts (not the feelings) of what is worrying you.
6. Remember, feelings are not facts.
7. Tell yourself (or your child) that nothing can be magically sorted, but that often with calm step-by-step attention, things can be made a lot better.
8. Brainstorm a diagram of options – realistic or not – beside each worry, then take a break, returning to delete what's not possible or to see what else has come up.
9. Remember there is no magic wand and sometimes life is just unkind – it doesn't mean you have to be unkind to yourself, too.

9. Expectation

This is the wishful thinking that fuels resentment, and is the biggest precursor to relapse, so worth learning to navigate. Expectations are the unrealistic 'shoulds' and 'if onlys' that set you up to feel sorry for yourself, to feel justified in your annoyance. But despite the validity of your claim, it's what you do with this that is crucial. What you don't want is for someone else's actions to dominate your life and it takes great maturity and self-discipline to make sure this doesn't happen, especially where there has been abuse of some kind.

There is nothing more normal than to expect to, for example, eat tonight or wake up tomorrow morning, but the kinds of 'expectation' that are really troublesome are the kind that litter everyday life, accumulating into an attitude of annoyance that primes you for the 'gravity drop' into blame and shame: 'if only my son would work harder (lazy s***)', 'my daughter shouldn't speak to me like that (rude b****) . . .'. Left unchecked this kind of wishful thinking will turn into a resentment where someone is to blame, and left unaddressed, over time will stick, potentially affecting development of their identity and self-esteem as a result of your negative view.

The best way to counter this is to challenge the specifics of the 'should'. Of course, you'd like your son to work more, but why doesn't he? Curiosity is the most effective antidote to offence. People accrue lots of these kinds of incidental negatives as a result of their shoulds and if onlys that mean that later on in the day or in the week they are ready to tip over the edge into rage.

Common resentments that I come across can be as seemingly petty as judging and criticising other people as they walk down pavements ('do you drive like that?'), join a queue ('who do you think you are? I was here before you') or while driving. Consider the self-righteous perception of a car which 'should not have pushed in' in that way so that to punish them, the other driver will flash, shout and threaten. This argument can easily develop into physical blows and it is born of expectation and the Drama Triangle of resentment, as articulated by Stephen Karpman almost forty years ago (see Chapter 8). Central in Transactional Analysis, a popular model in psychology that considers social interaction and behaviour through the lens of three main ego states – parent (critical/nurturing), adult (rational) and child (intuitive/dependent) – and acknowledges the influence of past events on current experience, the Drama Triangle poses three positions to take of persecutor, victim and rescuer. You can join two others to play out this pattern or engage in all three in your head. What is certain is that it is always someone's fault as the triangle circulates around blame and shame.

The key to better management of expectation is to spot it as it's happening, and do a reality check instead, being curious as to what their/your 'should' or 'if only' was, and whether it was actually possible. The first sign most people have that there is a resentment lurking, born of expectation, is a sense of disappointment and it is here that you must make the decision to either divert into curiosity and understanding, so that we may learn, or drop into the destructive conflict pattern that is resentment.

Actions:
Get yourself a small pad and a pen or pencil that will fit into your back pocket or bag and appoint a day in advance – stick to this date! On waking that day, I suggest you mark down how many times you say or think 'should', 'ought' or 'if only', as well as the negatives of each. Count how many times you engage in this wishful and judgemental thinking over a day. It's hard to do and some people tell me that they do a few hours and then multiply, but if you can, stick to it for a day. Most people are stunned by how their 'stinking thinking' and wishful thinking set them up for lots of the pain and resentment that they have otherwise thought was somebody else's fault.

10. Resentment

There are three main forms of anger: healthy anger, resentment and rage. Resentment is the smoldering anger that feeds on blame and fuels rage. The biggest precursor to relapse, resentment is 'drinking the poison and expecting the other person to suffer'; it's 'poor me', 'bad you' or 'bad me / poor you'. One of the most toxic relational patterns, resentment plays out through the Drama Triangle, a circuit of blame on other or on self (i.e. shame), a dead end, a trap whereby it's always someone's fault.

Families are prime territory for this pejorative relational pattern and although it may start in subtle ways (and some people reading this may recognise this as 'normal human behaviour'), when it develops into a relational pattern that relies on side-taking and conflict it can become dangerous. What needs to be respected and understood is that in 'victim', a person will feel they have a right to abdicate responsibility and in addiction terms that means relapse with impunity. In 'persecutor', a person will feel self-righteous in their belief of who is to blame – often displaying aggression and rage – and in 'rescuer', someone will feel compelled to come up with the answers, to soothe and to decide who is right and who is wrong. In fact, the rescuer is the person who makes the Drama Triangle complete as they decide who is victim and who is persecutor by who they give their support to. And in giving this support, in defending the victim, they take sides and show a lack of faith that the victim can take care of themselves.

It's definitely worth understanding resentment as a way of thinking and feeling that takes hostages, fuels blame and can split families so that love becomes distorted. It's worth understanding to prevent this from happening and to prevent yourself, as a parent, from inadvertently fuelling the self-destructive behaviour in your child that may later become apparent as an addictive process. There is simply no place for resentment in a healthy relationship.

> **Actions:**
> Pick a day for logging when you fall into victim (poor me), persecutor (bad you) or rescuer (urgent with answers for others) – a separate day for each.
> - Describe how one of each of these played out.
> - How did you feel in each example?
> - Did you think about how the other person felt?
> - Was the outcome productive/constructive?
> - What were your common themes, thoughts or feelings? Some common examples:
>   - People should do what I would do in that scenario.
>   - That's not polite.
>   - That's not fair.
>   - What about me?
>   - You're an idiot.
>   - Why do I have to do everything?
> - Explore at least one of these, all the way through asking yourself why at every answer.

11. Isolation

There are two distinct forms of isolation: one is being physically on one's own and the other is the emotional, psychological or even spiritual loneliness of not letting others connect.

Alone in a crowd, someone who suffers from the early stages of addiction can be surrounded by other people and even appear to be popular without ever feeling secure. They are more likely to focus on how they feel different and compare how they feel against how other people look, inevitably coming off worse.

. . . .

Janet came in worried about her daughter Keira, who was eleven years old. She said that she would ask Keira if she'd like having a friend over at the weekend and Keira would reply that she didn't have any friends. Worried, Janet had sought advice from the school, who were surprised, telling her that Keira was one of the most popular girls and always surrounded by friends. Janet had tried to tell her daughter this, but Keira repeatedly got angry and it had become a no-go subject between them. It seemed that despite her apparent popularity, Keira felt apart from the others, and it was her feelings that Janet had to learn to help Keira with, teaching that feelings weren't facts! So telling her that everyone could see she was surrounded by friends only served to make Keira feel more lonely. It wasn't until her mother acknowledged how painful that must be for Keira, despite their different perspectives, that Keira began to soften and let her in.

Such is the fear of being found out to be a fraud or a disappointment, young people will often defend against letting anyone genuinely connect with them. In addiction, when both of these forms of isolation combine, it usually creates a rock bottom with such a profound sense of loneliness that many people describe how it would be better to die.

What I've learned over my years as a therapist is that the isolation that happens where there is an absence of a kind relationship with yourself can be the most damaging. Once you have learned how to make yourself your own best friend you will never experience that kind of loneliness again.

As social creatures the sense of belonging is a core social motive that fractures isolation and allows us to connect and feel part of something. Sadly, the defence mechanisms that are so often triggered in childhood in order to feel safe can create a façade that leaves people hidden in plain view. Pretending you are not what you look like or that you don't think or feel what you do means that you deny your true self, and as a result cannot connect.

Questions:
- Are you fearful of letting people close to you?
- Do you know what this is about – what childhood experiences or messages have you taken on-board?
- Can you choose someone to trust and begin to tell them more about you?
- If you don't have anyone, can you see a therapist or attend a fellowship meeting and begin the process of connecting intimately (not meant in a sexual way)?
- Do you think your child is isolating?
- What's that like for you to witness? Try to manage your own feelings so you don't project them onto your child at this vulnerable time.
- What childhood experiences or messages do you think they have taken on-board?

Actions:
- From a place of calm self-respect, can you begin to inch towards talking to your child about what they believe? Don't argue with what they tell you about themselves – i.e. that they have no friends – listen, comment on what that must feel like, admit it's not necessarily what you see, but own that that doesn't mean what they're saying isn't true.
- Try not to fix the problem but instead ask them what they want to do about it and support them to find answers. In doing this, you're already fracturing their isolation and showing them that they won't be shamed or humiliated by letting someone in.

12. Self-centeredness/self-pity/self-will

In the fellowship rooms, alcohol-ISM is known as 'alcohol-I Self Me', and you can apply this across all the addictive processes as they are all totally self-centred, even if the behaviour is to self-neglect. In this fear-based relationship with the world, paradoxically, in order to feel safe, in control of others and of life, the addict has to be totally self-absorbed. Common to all addiction is a feeling of low self-worth and poor self-esteem, and this can often be coupled with a profound self-consciousness, heightened anxiety or even paranoia that everybody is looking, that the world is out to get you.

At the centre of their own world, leaving little space for any other people to be close to them, the person suffering from addiction will do everybody else's thinking for them and react accordingly before those around them even have a chance to make up their minds, let alone express what they think.

Operating from a negative core belief, the addict will often set up those around them to react to them in a certain way. So if the addict can't make you laugh and control how you see them in that way, they are likely to provoke you to dislike them. What's important is that they are in charge. The hypervigilance that this requires means that an addict can make a drama out of nothing, they will see something worth reacting to in every-thing – a wrong look, physical movement, a clumsy comment, all are enough to trigger an extreme response.

Running parallel to self-centeredness is the kind of self-will that if it were applied to achieving greatness or overcoming difficulty would be an asset worth having. The condition is known as self-will run riot: 'I want what I want and I want it now'. Although addicts may present with anxiousness and uncertainty, and many will even seek help or advice from other people, they are unlikely to actually follow through on the help that they get. Much more likely is a pattern of addicts seeking advice or talking about the troubles they have to friends or those they love, almost as a way of purging the discomfort instead of actually seeking practical change, preferring to defer to their own tried and tested techniques, no matter how dysfunctional.

But the emotional price of this kind of self-centred self-will is a profound sadness and loneliness, akin to feeling hopeless and helpless, that is self-pity. Almost everyone I've ever met who suffers from addiction claims to detest self-pity, all the while wallowing in a victim position that confirms a 'what's the point' attitude. This 'pity party' can kill, as when somebody gets it into the head that nobody cares, nobody can help and nobody wants to anyway then the drug of choice can really take hold as the best and only solution. 'Poor me, poor me . . . pour me another drink.'

As a parent, it is vital to proactively challenge this self-centeredness so that the child learns the other centered qualities that will allow them to feel part of a social network. Asking how others are and being interested comes from watching a parent do the same and from being affirmed for doing it themselves. Recognising other people have feelings and an agenda themselves that still allows space for that of others will help the child accept their own needs and wants as valid.

Most children are open to taking guidance on-board unless or until they are exposed to this in a negative form and then they will self-protect by being wilful (compliance or defiance). Listening to what your child feels they need or want, not always giving in, but always showing that you understand their view is important, followed by then standing shoulder to shoulder with them as you both assess the success or otherwise of the outcome.

Importantly the self-pity is not challenged by old-fashioned comments such as 'boys don't cry', 'don't cry or I'll give you something to cry about' or 'get a grip', as it shames the child just as they are potentially learning the line between unhealthy self-pity and healthy compassion for self. Remember it is only those people who do not care about themselves that can repeatedly do themselves damage.

Questions:
- When you offer to do something or want to say something, is it for you or for the other person's benefit?
- Do you give freely or is there often a catch?
- How willing is your child to help?
- When you ask your child to do something for you, do you ask them to 'do you a favour', or is helping part of the family culture? (If it's the former it will cause a lot of trouble and needs to stop!)

Actions:
- If your child appears selfish, and only takes care of him- or herself, perhaps you have either done too much for them in the past or perhaps they feel neglected and as a result are self-reliant. If this is the case, they will struggle to accept any help or input from the parent. In order to challenge these behaviours depending on their age, your approach must be compassionate and genuinely curious, firm but kind – and make sure you are being honest too as children are often very quick to point out hypocrisy!

- Think about who in your life you are prepared to trust, and commit to asking those people for advice when you don't know what to do, and then follow it. Allow them to help you – don't just ask, receive!

- If you are worried that your child suffers from self-will, ask yourself what it is about you that might make it hard for them to receive from you and work on it. Perhaps you are very opinionated so they lose their own mind if they involve you, or maybe you become overly worried. If your relationship with your child is good enough, ask them why they don't ask for your advice, though sometimes it is appropriate that a teen no longer asks their parents, but you would hope they are leaning on friends who have their best interest at heart. If they don't appear to, either you're misjudging the friends or your child is heading down the wrong road.

- Challenging someone in self-pity is hard as whatever you do will reinforce the victim state. Try to be genuine and show that you care, but admit that you don't have the answers. If your child is in self-pity, they will try to shame you for being so ineffective – just tell them that you care and that you can see they are hurting and that you are there for them. Remember this is a marathon not a sprint!

These twelve points that make up The Core Characteristics™ are compiled from my experience of being in recovery myself, from working with teams in therapeutic environments and from helping people come back from the living hell that is active addiction. They give us a vital focus for early intervention and prevention so that we can help our children to learn to be resilient and in good and esteemed self-knowledge, so they never need to self-medicate to such painful proportions.

The Core Characteristics™ are ordinary human qualities that if they become extreme in any way warrant immediate attention – with no negative side effects! Promoting well-being in parent and child, this model also validates the conscious integration of well-being and emotional intelligence in schools, where teachers are *in loco parentis*, as a priority.

Also, at the other end of the scale, even after the addiction has taken hold, a focus on addressing The Core Characteristics™ instead of making sobriety the goal means addiction doesn't have to be a chronic relapsing condition for everyone. Instead, being sober is the first step, as it removes the band aid, which can hurt and can feel very scary . . . very. It's worth remembering that if your child agrees to give up an addictive behaviour, you will feel proud and pleased – but they won't, not at first anyway.

It's unusual, too, for someone who develops addiction to have only one 'drug of choice' and this is called 'cross addiction'. As we've discussed, alcohol use is linked to a sweet tooth and weight gain; anorexia and bulimia are often linked to self-harm, exercise or shoplifting; codependence and overeating often come together. Sometimes, when the more obvious and worrying form of addiction is challenged and sobriety sought, another apparently less dangerous form can take its place, which parents often feel they have to put up with as the lesser of the two evils. If it's addiction your child is suffering from, then another addiction won't fix it. Instead, keep your eye on your child and notice how they treat themselves and others. This is where attention to The Core Characteristics™ can play a vital part.

Questions:
- How are you around The Core Characteristics™? What feelings do they bring up in you when you read about them?
- Do you notice yourself in any of them?
- Are you minimising and dismissing this thinking as pathologising normal human behaviours?
- What would be the harm in recognising and dealing with each of these?
- What might be the harm if you don't?
- Which ones are you worried about in your child?
- What does this bring up in you?

Just remember that you matter too – start with you so that what you say to your child has integrity and accepts that you are involved in some way in how they behave.

5

CODEPENDENCY

Surely codependency is just good manners?

A pattern of loving without loving yourself, many people are codependent without realising it and may cause harm that they later deeply regret. The point is to be able to give 'digested love' so that it comes from a place of profound self-love and self-respect, so that your giving is not hypocritical. As children, we must take from our parents and if we feel our parents can ill afford the time or energy, it will stop us from being able to reach out, no matter how 'lovely' or 'giving' our parents seem to be. Worse, it might set that child up to caretake the needs of the parent, thereby denying their own needs to devastating effect as they may repeat this pattern in all their relationships. Putting a name to this complex dimension of addiction sheds light on the experience of relationships that is essential for both parent and child.

It would be impossible, maybe even negligent, to address the subject of addiction without mentioning codependency in some detail, as wherever there is one, there is the other. Most people struggle to understand what codependence is (even if they are self-confessed codependents) and over the years it has become one of my specialised areas, in part because of my passion to really go the distance, into the corners, to give someone the best chance of recovery possible, as many people who suffer from addiction are also codependent. Some even think it is the root of all addiction. I have been personally affected by codependence all my life, in myself and in others I have been close to, and it has shaped me in ways I now regret as it took me a long time to learn how to recognise my needs and give them the appropriate time and attention rather than all or nothing, indulge neglect.

The way I describe codependency is 'conditional giving presented as unconditional giving'. It is 'don't worry about me, let's worry about you (now do you like me?)'. It is a way of life whereby as the codependent you are never the priority. You're the person who says 'no, it's alright, I'll be fine, let's focus on you' or who overlooks your own even most basic need to eat or to sleep, in favour of attempting to fulfil somebody else's wishes. All the people with whom I have worked who are codependent are running on empty because they don't know how to put fuel into their own tank. More than that, it feels wrong to prioritise self, almost shaming that they might actually have needs themselves.

Why codependence?

Let me explain. I had a nightmare as a child, a recurring dream . . .

. . . .

Floodwater surges through the high street, in the walls of the village shops, sucking at their foundations. The wheels of upturned cars protrude like gravestones, and bins and plastic bottles rush past me, pulled by the hidden current. People are screaming and I can see arms stretching up from the murky depths grasping for an anchor, a hand. I am in a rowing boat. The only boat in sight. I start to grab those hands. I am pulling people into my boat, shapeless, dark weights, heavy with water. There is no more room and the weight of the boat is heaving towards the corner where I realise there is a dangerous waterfall, a sheer drop, and we are heading straight for it. The boat is heavy, full. There is no more room. I look down into the swirling water, yellowish green and thick. I have to anchor the boat to something. I am the only one who can do this. I jump in. The water is cold and I can feel it pulling at me, urging me under. I go with it and dive deep into the shadows. I am holding a rope and in my mind I see a

streetlight. I dive blind until I feel the smooth, slender shape of the
curve before the bulb, and I tie the rope. The boat is secure. I let go. I
feel myself fall deep, deep into the darkness, pulled into the power of
the flood, sucked away, and I cannot fight. I am gone.

As I considered this dream with the help of a therapist, I realised that the self-imposed role of saviour had become a trap for me, so that I sought out crisis or created drama in every relationship. The strain made me volatile and intense and was powerfully self-defeating, isolating me from the connection I longed for. Letting the role go helped me to calm down, and it also left space for another version of Mandy to evolve. As I got into recovery and challenged the thinking that I was 'the only one who' could save the world (my family?), this nightmare subsided and I have not had it now for nearly twenty years.

Where does codependence come from?

The child that experiences a parent or sibling in constant high need will also be likely to witness the impact that has on the rest of the family in terms of emotional and time resources. The child might still demand attention and time, but is increasingly aware of the strain on those who might take care of him or her. As a result, that child makes a decision based on survival that will change their life – 'if I don't need, then I won't add to the strain, which will then make things safer around here'. Instead of needing, the child becomes the good girl or the good boy, contributing to the system, by 'good' behaviour, e.g. washing their hands before supper (without being told to), coming when they are called (first time), doing their prep without being nagged, and by being caring, e.g. always asking the parent if they are OK or if they need a hug. They are rewarded by being told things like 'you're my good girl/boy, where would I be without you?' This reward causes that child to commit to this way of being, neglecting their own needs in favour of 'people-pleasing' and gaining their sense of worth through external validation. Those early years set an almost unconscious foundation of experience in the world, providing a vital template around what that child expects and understands, and how they learn how to be. Often I meet people in their adulthood who describe feeling almost psychic in their ability to read the room, to read people's feelings and to understand a 'vibe'. This always requires gentle exploration to find out what it might have been that made it so necessary for that person to be so painfully aware. Even if they have turned this ability into an asset it's important to have done the work to disentangle the skill from the originating trauma. Having a violent father, for example, or an alcoholic mother or a self-destructive sibling can very quickly teach you how to read a room before you even walk into it, just so you know how to position yourself and survive.

The early years form a basic foundation for each child to interact with the world from. Where there is codependency I would describe this effect as a profound abandonment of self whereby although you can help others, and seem to be very effective at telling others what they're feeling and what they should do, you will find it almost impossible to identify your own feelings or to give them attention. The problem is that it can be hard to see the enormous price you pay for your people-pleasing.

I recently met a girl who had been present at one of my PSHE talks several years earlier. She said that she had thought I was overdoing it when I spoke of the dangers of codependence at the talk as she had loved being needed by others. But then when she failed to get into university because of low grades for her A levels, as a direct result of putting others' needs first, she regretted not listening more closely. It was a chance meeting, and she had just completed her retakes, but I was grateful for the reminder of how hard the reality of the codependent message is to hear. Helping others is socially affirmed and easy to fall into as a relational pattern, but abandon your own needs at your peril.

Often people are fearful of upsetting the codependent so they aren't honest with them. As a result of the lack of genuine interaction, the intimacy is inauthentic. This works the other way around too so that the codependent cannot give honest feedback and often says yes when they mean no, hiding the resentment they feel as a result. It's a terribly isolated place to live.

* *

Liza was in her early thirties. She remembered distinctly a moment in her childhood when she felt her codependency was activated. She described how she and her mother were going to do some cooking, she was about six or maybe seven years old. She had gone to get the baking tray, scales, mixing bowl out. She remembered with emotion that she had her own apron and was able to describe the stitch detail on the front. While she was preparing the ingredients, her mother nipped upstairs to see her brother, who Liza recalls as 'always angry'. He was older than her. Liza remembered hearing shouting upstairs and the door being slammed and then she watched as her mother came through the door of the kitchen, leaning against the doorjamb for a moment before turning around and viewing Liza with all her cooking things laid out on the kitchen table in preparation. Liza wasn't sure which came first, but she was able to clearly identify a look of what she felt was annoyance on her mother's face and a sense of embarrassment in her own chest. Working with me, Liza was able to later explore this emotion as shame. Her mother approached her and said that she didn't have time to do the cooking today and could Liza be a good girl and just put everything away and lay the table instead, as that would be really helpful; they would do cooking tomorrow. The sorrow Liza connected to in the session with me was profound. This was not her mother's fault, her brother's fault or even her own fault, but rather a consequence of something so common in family life, whereby one person's overt need trumps the rest. Like the cuckoo in the nest that grows and pushes the other eggs and birds out so that it can monopolise parental care, it is all too easy to divert attention and resources to the most obvious and critical need which may become addiction in its most recognisable form. This then justifies and reinforces that need as valid, and by default creates neglect elsewhere.

Whenever I meet an addict, I look for the sibling who is codependent. It would be negligent not to.

Why do you help like you do?

It is useful when working with addiction (or trying to take proactive steps to prevent it) to look for patterns and this is no exception. Notice if it is always the same person who gives up their needs and wants in favour of the family or another person, as if that is their role (identity). Liza had initially approached me to work on her relationship with her husband, who she described as selfish, and yet felt bad saying so. Through this work, we were able to trace how Liza had been primed in early childhood not to need. This was to compensate for her brother's overt emotional demands on her mother. Sadly, Liza had witnessed the emotional price her mother had paid for this and so found it impossible to want anything from her. In fact, Liza felt ashamed for wanting anything at all from her mother as she could see her mother was running on empty so she learned to prop her up by being a 'good girl'. We could follow the thread all the way through from that point in her childhood through primary school where she got consistently good reports about being helpful, reliable, always doing tidy-up time and often helping the new child to orientate. But when Liza hit secondary school, she fell in with a 'bad crowd'.

A bad crowd?

It's an interesting phrase and not one I particularly believe in. However it's a common belief and one which I hear about in the context of people like Liza, when their parents describe exactly the same scenario whereby the child has been super good all their lives until they hit secondary school, where they make friends with people who are troubled. These parents are bewildered, worried and feel completely out of their depth with this child they suddenly feel they don't know. I have to ask them a difficult question which is this: 'what happened to your daughter or your son, perhaps when they were seven or under, that meant that they know who to be and how to behave around difficult people and circumstances?'

Helping is who I am

The answer, of course, is that people like Liza will always gravitate towards people who need them to be selfless (quite literally), and focused on helping others, who present with such high needs that the Lizas of this world are constantly employed in caretaking, something which is both familiar and isolating, because that is all they know. Remember the wash of embarrassment or shame that swept through Liza when she saw her mum's regret that she had committed to doing the cooking? It is that moment, not as a one-off, but rather within a culture of reinforcement of the same message, that defines the codependent, setting them up to avoid being seen to need for the rest of their life. And this extends beyond needing help or care and attention into being unable to receive a compliment or an affirmation, and feeling embarrassed if somebody gives you a gift.

Spotting codependence as a priority

When I go into a school to talk about addiction or drugs and alcohol, I often ask the year group who among them has got a problem with drinking or with taking drugs, and my enquiry is invariably met with derision. But I am one step ahead. I then ask who among the group is the rock, the confidant, the one you can rely on to be there for you when you go through something difficult or when there's a drama or a crisis? I notice a few teens shift self-consciously in their seats and maybe three or four people out of a hundred will look at me as if to confirm that they know who they are. This is when I tell them that it is the people they are closest to, those high-maintenance friends, who are at risk of developing addiction in its most recognisable form, and that they are the secret keepers. I ask them, what is your payoff?

Challenging the codependency in a school year group, in an office or in the original social group that is the family are significant moves that can be made in cleaning them up emotionally. The codependent will be the secret keeper and thereby, without even realising it, often prevents the person who is struggling from accessing the professional help they may need. The codependent is the emotional shock absorber, preventing that person from experiencing the consequences and therefore learning from them and developing resilience. Codependence takes root in childhood and carries all the way through so it can manifest in a teen but just as easily in a parent, where it can easily hide behind the parental obligation of caretaking. The codependent is the person who will pick up the pieces, who will soothe you and be there for you in your darkest hour, but for many people who suffer from addiction dumping on a codependent enables them to go out and use again.

But the blame does not lie with codependents, as they are not responsible for the pain another might feel – far from it. I am suggesting that codependency warrants just as much attention as the classic addict. In my view and experience, codependency is the socially acceptable face of addiction, posing as love, care and other centredness. The motivation and the codependence, of which they are so often completely unconscious, is actually the self-centered motivation born of emotional starvation. *If I can anticipate your need and make you feel better, am I worthwhile? Will you love me?* A true dichotomy in other words, whereby your drug of choice is somebody else's problem because it makes you feel needed and validated, so you gravitate towards people who demand that you give. But if they get better, you are out of a job and if they love you, you can't take it in!

So who am I codependent on?

A popular myth that confuses people's ability to really take responsibility for the codependence that they might suffer from is to assume that they are codependent on one person in particular. This assumes that you can only be codependent if you have someone who is a qualifying addict that you are close to as if they cause your codependence. Instead the addict and the codependent will seek each other out.

The concept of codependency was first couched around 1951 when Al-Anon (the fellowship for families of alcoholics) formed, sixteen years after Alcoholics Anonymous, but it was in the 1980s that it was really recognised as a condition in its own right. Significantly codependency was thus first noticed in the partners of the addict or the alcoholic but then, in order to access the help that can change the codependent's life, the addict has to be identified.

Even in my own industry, if I ring up and speak to a therapist to refer a codependent for therapy, more often than not even that therapist will ask me who my client is codependent on. Of course, the simplicity of the term codependency is that the codependent lives in association with, as a support team to, in reflection of someone else and that someone else must remain in crisis or need to enable the codependent to have to give. Imagine the terror of the caretaker when the object of care starts to get well or to become independent. They are redundant, out of a job, perhaps they will be rejected or, worse, the focus might fall onto them, which will feel shameful and wrong. Thus a true codependent will surround themselves with people who are troubled, in high demand or important in some way, or in environments of crisis and drama which aid the codependent to put their needs to one side. Equally they might find one or two people in their lives who present with unusually high need, which could be emotional, mental health or physical, but which crucially lures the codependent into a caretaking role which they are then obliged to fulfil.

Simply codependency is the profound neglect of self that is powerfully enabled by seeking out people who demand that you neglect yourself. A true codependent will have more than one high-maintenance individual in their life. They may have their primary candidate but they will also have a way of life that perfectly fits the dysfunctional puzzle shape that they are.

· ·

If we go back to Liza, she had grown up in her brother's shadow, she had stood back from making demands on the family, her best friend at school had suffered from self-harm and she had fallen in love with a man who some would describe as narcissistic. Liza was also a PA to a CEO who was an extremely difficult man and she was exhausted by her work, but proud that he relied on her so

heavily. To really unpick the patterns whereby she had interwoven
herself into others lives as 'the prop' was painful. She realised that
she had significant responsibility for the very behaviours she was
complaining about, and for the experience of exhaustion and near
burnout that had brought her to my consulting room. In recognising
responsibility she now had the opportunity to change something.
That guilty feeling that had long since plagued Liza of 'what about
me' was about to get some proper airtime and attention.

Codependency is in my view one of the hardest conditions to get well from because it is like an emotional anorexia whereby psychopathologically in order to survive, the codependent decides that they do not need. Recovery is accepting that they do need and learning how to trust and receive nurture from others and from the world at large. This can often feel self-indulgent, self-centred, greedy and it can also feel terrifying as there may be a core belief that their need is greater than the sustenance on offer. But healthy selfishness is a skill worth learning as it allows you to have the capacity to be generous. Where a person feels that being caring is a natural interest and skill, that person is in my view obliged to learn how to take care of that skill and invest in inherent patterns of self-care so that they can be generous from a place of abundance, and so that their giving is unconditional. That means if the codependent (in recovery!) comes to help you, you don't have to be helped, if they offer comfort, you can receive it yet still feel sad. It means the codependent can enjoy giving and then let go.

Being the child of a codependent

My clients range in age from sixteen years upwards. Working with young people is always exciting because I believe that the sooner you can intervene upon an addictive process, the more positive and sustainable the potential outcome, and also less damage has been done. I even believe in a cure. But working with the under twenties demands that the family be involved for the most effective outcomes to be possible. This is because there is often still contact, a practical dependence and interaction on a frequent basis that remains a core influence to that young person's experience and way of life. So often in working with someone young who presents with an addictive process, it's clear that the addiction extends way beyond their acting out behaviour and into the family dynamic.

It should not be a surprise to us that addiction comes from the family greenhouse, the culture within which that person grew up and that working with the family in therapy is essential for effective treatment – ever more so when the 'addict' is a teenager. But I often meet with resistance as the family, perhaps unintentionally, scapegoat the 'addict' as the problem and therefore make them deserving of all the attention and financial/time resources, instead of allowing a process to unfold, whereby they are also involved. Counter-intuitively though, when the family take some of the responsibility they reclaim at least some of the power. For if one person is the whole problem, they are also the whole solution. Nothing comes out of nothing and children who have a codependent parent have their own dynamic to understand.

. . . .

A favourite story that I tell to illustrate this point is 'the cake story'. Katie recalls feeling like she was a monster through her childhood because everybody thought her mother was such a good, kind and lovely person, but Katie found her intensely irritating (despite also loving her). For many years, Katie recalled feeling that there was something wrong with her because she couldn't bear her mother's care, finding it controlling and suffocating as she offered unsolicited advice. Katie would often react aggressively to even the mildest of her mother's suggestions. She described as an older teenager visiting her mother, who by then had divorced her father. She arrived at the door and her mother opened it, delighted to see her and inviting her in for a cup of tea. Katie refused the tea, but her mother went ahead and made it anyway, all the while checking with her as to how she liked it, if it were the right colour, etc. Katie recalls getting ever more exasperated with this experience so that when her mother offered to give her some cake to go with her tea, her responses got shorter and shorter as her mother was ever more insistent in finding that piece of cake that Katie could have. Eventually Katie erupted, shouting – 'I DON'T WANT CAKE'. Then seeing her mother's hurt, she gave in, snatched the cake and aggressively put the tea and cake down on the table. At this point, her mother became concerned and moved to sit near Katie to tell her that she was very worried about Katie, given her temper. However, working with me, Katie came to realise that her irritation was that she had come to see her mother, but her mother had put tea and cake in the way. That the real irritation was born of the desperation in Katie that she was being given a mixed message, as she explained to me: 'Do you have any idea of what it is like to have a mother who does not have the self-esteem to know that her daughter comes to see her and has to put tea and cake in the way?'

. . . .

The irritation that Katie describes here is common in children who have a parent who is codependent. I have sat in many sessions where the child (most often the daughter to the mother) says that she needs her mother to prioritise her own needs so the daughter can take from her without feeling guilty, and the mother's answer is: 'I don't understand, but of course I will if that will help you. I just want you to be happy.' At which point, the daughter generally becomes exasperated and turns to ask me to help, if I can see what's going on. The mother then appears utterly bewildered. Of course, the key lies in the modelled behaviour which here is often such a mixed message: I want you to be happy (but I don't make sure I am happy); I want you to take (but I will only give). The work is to help the mother to be in such good self-care that she can offer to her daughter without needing anything back. Not even her daughter's happiness.

The children of the codependent often describe being told, for example, not to be angry, or *'please don't be sad'* in what might seem like caring and loving responses to an expression of what might be called negative or difficult emotion. But the overarching result is that the child: a) becomes fearful of these emotions as they learn that they shouldn't be having them (often this is the parent's own displaced fear of emotion); b) becomes inexperienced in these emotions so as they gain natural momentum yet remain unexpressed they demand greater forms of compensation; c) becomes disconnected from their emotions as they are unable to express them and learn from them as they grow up; or d) becomes 'emotionally agoraphobic' to stop showing spontaneous emotion for fear of someone meddling with them as soon as they are expressed. Instead, they will express 'false emotion' in such a way as to keep everyone happy without becoming vulnerable. This leads to a loss of sense of self and makes teenagers very angry, but also feel guilty as they hide who they are from the person who they should be closest to.

Being the partner of a codependent

I think it is always useful to reflect on where you might stand in this toxic relationship pattern. Are you codependent? If so, your partner will be demanding or high maintenance, or maybe it's the other way around. How does this impact your child? And if your child is codependent, then they will attract difficult people into their lives so they are obliged to caretake and do what they have learned to be good at. If this is the case, then the likelihood is that someone in the family is a high-maintenance individual or even willing to identify as an addict. If it is you, then you will have somehow struck up an unconscious deal with your codependent partner whereby you act out and they pick up the pieces. At times the roles will reverse, but you will predominantly inhabit one of the two roles as your relationship default setting. As a result, you will inevitably find your partner unbelievably supportive, loyal despite being treated badly or taken for granted, but also suffocating and controlling. You will not find anyone as loyal as a codependent, your 'wing man (or woman)', but it comes with a price. Woe betide you if you betray this contract. You will find that they anticipate your need (which you like), that they do most of the dirty work (which you like), but that somehow you feel obliged to them (which you begrudge) and they frequently want to have 'heavy' conversations that drag up the past (which you dread). But you must understand that they will not choose you as a partner (consciously or otherwise) if they do not feel there is work to be done on you.

Being the codependent

Then here is the news: YOU MATTER! Simple as that! But if you are codependent, this will feel very uncomfortable. In fact, not only uncomfortable, but counter-intuitive and fundamentally wrong. Most people reply smiling that they know they matter, that they have good self-care, that they appreciate my attention but that the real priority here is the child or partner and that if that person they're worried about is better, that's all they need. 'You're only ever as happy as your unhappiest child' is the prison so many parents report ruefully from, as if I will understand or even agree. I don't. I believe you are free to be as happy as you want to be, irrespective of circumstance; although some peoples' circumstances are harder than others, it is possible.

In fact, it's true to say that many a codependent parent has genuinely saved the life of their troubled child as crisis management is what they are best at. But what they struggle to see, and therefore to change, is how their behaviour towards themselves, as much as to anyone else, has contributed to the pain that fuels that very crisis. This material is often found in the simplest of domestic tasks, such as tidying up the house, doing the shopping or preparing a meal. While the codependent resentfully peels and chopped carrots in the kitchen (alone again while the others are laughing and watching TV), picks up all the washing (while the others demand an ironed shirt) or goes once again to the shop for that vital ingredient (because no one else can be bothered), they will be feeling angry and resentful that they are the only person who seems to see this mess, do this job or even care. When somebody pops their head round the door and offers help though, the codependent is prone to refusing the help, saying 'it's OK, I've nearly finished'. On questioning, many people who suffer from codependency will explain that it is just quicker and easier to do the job themselves, displaying a distrust in other people's ability and a resistance to admitting they'd like help as if there was something wrong in that.

The subsequent resentment that boils just beneath the surface of a codependent experience of life can cause extreme ill health, stress, burnout and mental breakdown. But they will resist help until they have no fight left. Too often I meet people who are codependent about to lose their jobs, marriages and in dangerous ill health. I wish you would seek help for yourself sooner!

Patterns of rescue

As the codependent comes to the rescue, they create good/bad; right/wrong and inadvertently reinforce the very blame and shame they seek to avoid. Rescue creates a victim and enables the rescuer to self-neglect all the while looking like they know what needs to change in the other people or person. Think about that. I have known many parents and partners who have paid off the debt of their loved one who is an addict, relieving the financial consequence and then feeling resentful that the addict goes out and spends again.

If you are a natural caretaker, and you are kind and loving as a person and want to share this ability and these qualities, it is my firm belief that you have a responsibility to first ring-fence these assets by learning to be kind and caring to yourself, so that you may give from a place of nourishment. One well-known example is when on an aircraft if the plane goes into crisis, and the oxygen masks drop down, you are well advised to put the oxygen mask over your face first so that you can go on to (safely and effectively) help others. This is a great analogy for what a codependent in recovery must learn to do, despite it going against the grain. But when you give from a place of exhaustion and need to be acknowledged and when you're running on empty, your care is more likely to come across as control, as if the person you have helped is obliged to feel better, to be helped 'after all you've done for them'. You will feel a need for the person to experience a positive result of your intervention or support. You will be waiting for a score, a well done, a 'we couldn't have done it without you', a validation.

A true codependent will deny this as you are not even allowed to privately believe you need to receive the validation you so deeply crave. And, of course, therefore resentment will follow: 'after all I've done for you and you treat me like that'.

If you are codependent and are reading this chapter, you may feel uneasy, angry even, at the suggestion that a lot of your giving to others is in fact conditional, that you want something back and that you feel so unappreciated and resentful.

I remember very clearly being in treatment myself and sitting up all night talking to a fellow in my group. I listened to him for hours, despite myself needing sleep and time to reflect on my own process. I sat and worked out what it was that was hurting him, where he needed to focus and what he could do to really help himself. When we went into group therapy the next day, he opened the group with all these revelations of what he had worked out, where his focus needed to be and what his intended course of action was. As he sat there smiling, receiving affirmation from the rest of the group, I knew I was waiting for him to say 'I couldn't have done this without Mandy, she's the one who helped me'. But it never came. I felt so angry that day with him; it was only my trust in the group that allowed me to have the revelation I needed several days later when I expressed how I felt; I could have better spent my time focusing on myself instead. As he said to me that day, words that so many of you who are codependent will recognise: 'Everybody benefits from you, Mandy, except you. Think about that.' I did, I do.

In this simple experience we find the abiding features of the codependent which strangely lie in an apparently instinctive capacity to rescue, having good ideas about finding answers around other people's difficulties, around problem-solving. But crucially what a codependent can do for others, they cannot do for themselves. Everybody benefits from the codependent except the codependent themselves and the backlash is that the codependent is often described as suffocating and controlling.

So, if you do identify with these descriptions, there will be answers here for you because removing that thread of resentment born of the inability to value yourself sets your caretaking free to be giving without condition. It will allow you to really take care of yourself and of the capacity you have to care about others, to really learn how to better manage that skill as a valuable asset in your repertoire.

Questions:

- Are you better at giving or receiving?
- What are the feelings for you when you give?
- What are the feelings for you when you receive?
- Notice if you feel any power or strong sense of worth when you give – what do you think it's like to receive from you?
- Notice if you feel distrustful or obliged when you receive – what do you think it is it like to give to you?
- Do you accept you have needs and wants? How do you meet them?
- How committed are you to self-care, even if not in an overt way?
- Does your child struggle to receive, preferring instead to give to others?
- How do they suffer as a result?
- Do they put others' needs ahead of their own?
- Can you begin to model a healthier pattern of behaviour to them in relation to others so that they can begin to learn to give from a place of nourishment and good self-esteem?

Actions:

- Attend the CoDA fellowship (see The Essentials on page 221).
- Talk to your child about how important it is to learn to take care of yourself so you can afford to be generous with others. Perhaps point out that some of the worries they are having about others are: i) distracting them from their own life, and ii) enabling that person not to take responsibility for themselves. Don't forget that rescue creates a victim!

ADULT CHILD OF THE ALCOHOLIC (ACOA)

Most alcoholics are at work

I prefer the acronym to represent the Adult Child of the Addicted family system, so this is no longer just about alcohol as it was when the condition was first identified, it's about addiction, whatever the drug of choice. Once you recognise addiction as extreme self-destructive behaviour(s) that stem from unresolved pain and which perpetuate self-loathing, then it doesn't take much to appreciate how damaging it would be to grow up in an environment of active addiction. This is about those children who suffer because their parents suffer.

If you are a parent who is ACoA, your achievement is likely to be measured in terms of how different you are to your own parents. But no one gets off scot-free from a childhood steeped in addiction. I outline roles later in this chapter that people fall into as a result. It's likely to affect how you interact with others, your sense of identity and esteem and crucially how you parent yourself even if your hope is to be the opposite of what you experienced. To become conscious of how your own childhood shaped you, appreciating this in more detail, will allow you to consider your decisions as a parent that reflect who you are and not who you were primed to be. It will also help you to genuinely make sure that you do not repeat the painful patterns from your own childhood.

In order to proactively parent to prevent addiction, you cannot be in active addiction yourself. Even getting help but not accepting the status of being an addict or alcoholic can indicate shame that blocks full recovery. It's a family condition and I believe that the children deserve to know at an age-appropriate time about the sickness that travels through their family, and also be taught that recovery is possible.

Experience tells me that the kind of dysfunctional behaviours commonly found in the addictive family system can also be found in families where there are physical disabilities or mental health conditions like depression, anxiety or AD(H)D that negatively affect the family's ability to function healthily. The stigma of addiction prevents many people from accessing the benefits of the understanding and the wisdom held by so many in recovery themselves, or by those who have dedicated their lives and their careers to treating this condition. If you can get over that stigma you can access the wealth of information that can help, and it should not cause any harm either.

Why ACoA?

Recognition of the ACoA experience was first noted in the early 1980s (Wegscheider-Cruse, 1980; Black, 1981; Woititz, 1983; Middleton-Moz, 1985) and quickly grew in popularity. Almost overnight all those people who had previously lived holding their breath, with an unnamed feeling of shame that went so far back it felt like it *was* who they were, found out there was a reason they felt like they did. In her 1983 book *Adult Children of Alcoholics*, Janet G. Woititz speaks about the experience of being the (adult) child of the alcoholic, validating the term. Nowadays we know a lot more about this experience, although in the UK it is not as well attended to in the treatment field, and certainly not in the medical profession, as in the United States, and this needs to change.

It is even harder to recognise the impact of addiction on the rest of your family than it is to identify an addict, and that's not easy. The social stigma of identifying yourself with the pejorative term of addict or alcoholic in a world where there is so little understanding (in my view) of the true nature of addiction means that in standing up and being counted, that in asking for help, you potentially take on a whole load of negative projections of being e.g. weak, immoral or bad. So, instead, you opt for denial and explain away the clues and symptoms as one-offs. But in my view owning that you are an addict of any kind gives you the choice to either use it as an excuse, or to take responsibility, and as a therapist and a recovering addict myself, I encourage the latter. As the saying goes, 'you are as sick as your secrets', and for the child of the addict, the secret they keep is not theirs, so being honest relieves that burden at least.

It is so very, very hard for a family member to bring a concern about a loved one's drinking to a professional forum as it makes it real. So hard that most people miss the opportunity of early intervention so that by the time they arrive in my office there are severe consequences already in place.

What is alcoholism? When does anything become an addiction?

If you consider alcoholism to be about how much somebody drinks, then perhaps in weighing up their drinking against their earning or career you might decide that 'it's not that bad'. Tragically what doesn't usually happen in this assessment of someone's drinking is thinking about the family or the children at home – and the inevitable relational vacuum that is intrinsic in addiction which prevents healthy close and intimate relationships. There is a behaviour in place (alcohol) that compensates for an emotional need (e.g. stress, self-esteem issues, fear of intimacy) that has become a need in its own right (continued drinking) so that this emotional need remains hidden in the real world. Consider the alcoholic to be someone suffering from all The Core Characteristics™ of addiction, somebody who is profoundly and viscerally resistant to vulnerability, so that the prospect of connection triggers a fear of being hurt, then we are looking at somebody who cannot connect emotionally in a healthy way. Thus I believe the term 'functional alcoholic' (or addict) to be a dangerous oxymoron and it should be struck from our professional rhetoric. There is no such thing.

Imagine what it is to be their child, with a parent who might look successful or functional, but who suffers from low self-esteem, who doesn't really feel as if they are there. Or who seems to choose work over the family time and time again. And that's at best. For many more, the parent is not only 'not there' but they are also volatile and in too many cases, the child becomes an obvious target to displace this feeling against as they cannot effectively defend themselves.

Children of 'functional alcoholics'

Often scapegoated into addictive behaviour themselves, the children of so-called 'functional alcoholics' arrive mutinous in my office, often with a parent wringing their hands, bemoaning their loss of potential. When these children start talking, they are angry. They have often been given money to fix their emotional needs as it is the currency that enables the parent to feel functional. They have been placed second to the drinking. They often see their parent as a hypocrite. But crucially they are also often protective of the parent, and this creates considerable internal conflict which, in turn, can prompt a need to self-medicate in their own way. The lies and secrets that they have been silently asked to keep so that the alcoholic status quo can remain hidden has left them with no alternative but to act out (or act in).

Welcome to the world of the adult child of an alcoholic. Self-sufficient yet insecure, these children also often feel guilty about their feelings of anger and sense of neglect as they can see their parent is not well. The parent often feels afraid of the child as there is an unspoken power shift where the child knows the parent's Achilles heel. This can create a bullying approach by the parent or an enmeshing one, but either way the child will almost certainly distance themself from the parent, creating profound loss that they may not even be aware of immediately.

How is addiction in your family?

Addiction travels through families and across generations as addiction begets addiction. Sometimes it is highly visible, such as in the case of alcoholism, and sometimes less so if you consider the harder to spot addictive processes such as eating disorders, sex and love addiction, shopping or work. But in all these cases, there will be a profound avoidance of being emotionally available alongside a resentful and self-destructive relationship with self and with the world. Having read the chapter on The Core Characteristics™, you will now be aware of the distorted human qualities that lie beneath any addictive process.

Childhood is the 'greenhouse' in which we grow and develop into who we are; it's where we take root and develop our attachment process – i.e. who we are in relation to the world. With addiction, there are usually volatile mood, secrecy, shame, resentment and rage as constants and these will impact the child in terms of their relationship with others and also themselves – they will completely shape their life and compromise spontaneity and self-esteem.

One of the reasons addiction travels so easily in families is because we neither recognise nor treat the wider impact in the relational dimension that is codependency and the adult child of the addict. The codependent, as we have already learned in Chapter 4, is the 'perfect partner' for the addict, and the ACoA can often become an addict or codependent themselves. Often realising these profiles can 'carry' the addiction into the next generation, unwittingly, in their denial and desire not to be like their parent, they generate the same dynamic for themselves all over again, but this time it's with their own children.

To recognise this in advance is to open up a priceless opportunity for early intervention. Given my own background of acting out behaviour, I was excruciatingly attuned to any negative similarity between my children and me. It was a primary teacher who gave me this almost as a throwaway comment, and I've never forgotten it: **'Your child is not you. He doesn't have the same parents as you'**. In that moment, I realised that everything could be different.

Where do you get your parenting style from?

Certainly our children teach us how to be parents, but so do our parents. If you are repeating the patterns from your own parents, are you happy with this, or are you unaware of it? Perhaps you have determined to parent differently, aiming for the opposite without realising that if you do you are still driven by the same stimuli that were your parents. It is always interesting for us as parents to consider our own childhoods to see what is influencing how we parent our children, and to maintain an attitude of self-reflection that fosters empathy in our interactions with our children.

It's valuable to consider a dynamic such as ACoA because it recognises the influence of the environment that a child grows up in in terms of their development. Thus a parent can look back on the childhood environment of their offspring and retrospectively understand why their child is behaving as they are, and feel more patient with that understanding as they recognise their part in it. Better still when the soon-to-be parent has sufficiently good knowledge of themselves so they know how their own childhood might affect their own parenting. This will allow them to initiate boundaries or raise awareness to prevent some of the negative patterns repeating from the outset.

The goal is to be constructive. Remember, it's never too late.

Questions:
- Were you brought up with a lot of structure or were you left to your own devices?
  - What impact does this have on your experience of structure?
- Did you find either parent very controlling?
  - What impact does this have on how you do or don't seek to control your own child?
- Was there any violence in your family as you grew up?
  - What impact does this have on your experience of conflict?
- Did anyone in your family demand a lot of attention or have an addiction?

o   What impact did this have on your feelings about
     addiction or drugs and alcohol or attention-seeking
     behaviour?
- Which role do you feel you played as a child?
- Do you feel compelled to repeat that role now?
    o   How does that affect your parenting now?
    o   What impact does that have on your perception of yourself
         as a parent?

The common consequences of ACoA

1. Hypervigilance

Simply growing up in an environment of active addiction is to live on tenter-
hooks, waiting for the next drama and, in order to survive, the child must
become hypervigilant. This hypervigilance is required to survive such a
volatile environment and is a form of post-traumatic stress disorder (PTSD).
As someone gets older, this sensation is something that some describe as
being psychic, by others as being especially intuitive or being able to read
people. But as they engage in the therapeutic work, they begin to realise
that this skill has been born of a need to survive. They have learned to read
the parent from a tip of the shoulder, a change in tone, a twitch of brow
and crucially they had learned how to adjust so as not to inflame anything.

2. Intensity-seeking

When what is familiar is extreme or intense emotional experience, it is hard
to turn down that emotional thermostat and find something less intense
attractive. If you think about a child helpless and vulnerable aged seven,
eight or nine years old, exposed to a raging parental attack because they
spilled their drink or made a noise, what impact do you think that has on
that child when that happens repeatedly? When yesterday a noise triggered
an attack, but today it was ignored? Then maybe in the morning that parent,
full of remorse, seeks to compensate for their behaviour so is affectionate,

friendly, without acknowledging how they have behaved. Imagine how that child tries to make sense of that experience where any single move can make things worse. Imagine the terror that home is so unpredictable and frightening. If you can imagine these things, it will make sense that lots of those children learn how to dissociate, almost leave their own bodies as a form of self-protection. This extreme relational experience sets the template for future relationships, whereby in adulthood the child will not be able to tolerate a quiet norm as it will feel threatening. As it is familiar, the ACoA seeks out and often creates high drama and intense situations and relationships that demand they stay in the adrenalised state.

3. Hypersensitivity

Often the target of displaced emotion and projections, the child of the addict will have been exposed to unfair, disrespectful and often abusive behaviour from the very people who should be there to protect him or her. Blamed and scapegoated as the problem and yet, at the same time, responsible for making everything better, this child will be super sensitive to any suggestion of blame. At school, there is no resilience to playground banter and competitive jostling; in friendship, there is a fear of getting close in case the friend discovers the shameful secret and, in adulthood, even in marriage, where you may think there is some security, the hint of criticism can trigger unwarranted defensiveness – and a jokey slight can be easily misinterpreted and cause offence, resulting in sulking and a dark mood that can go on for days. It's tragic really because this child so misrepresents themselves, pushing away the love they so crave.

4. Control

As they had no control over their environments as a child, the ACoA will learn to control whatever they can within it. Thus a common reaction to feeling controlled is to seek control in another way, commonly through compliance or defiance. I believe that people who are very controlling are often people who experienced being controlled in a way that was terrifying, so they compensate and make sure it never happens again.

Compliance is the good child who never causes a stir or upsets anyone, always seeking to control everyone's mood by soothing or caretaking, always seeking to control what you think of him or her by being perfect. Defiance is the provoker: as a result of the lack of control over something abusive happening, the defiant child seems to invite it, in coming across as provocative, but is actually terrified and just controlling what they can – i.e. the timing of the abuse. In their shame-based belief that there is something wrong with them (to deserve the abuse from the parent), they get there first, setting you up to reject them / be scared of them / call them difficult / treat them like a monster – and in this defence they are all alone.

5. Self-reliance

Having been let down so profoundly by the original authority figures, children grow up distrusting their parents can properly advise and guide them, so revert to working things out for themselves, wholly relying on themselves. Often this child will have been affirmed for being so independent, and many go on to apply this distrust to all systems and authority figures, becoming entrepreneurs, politicians or leaders who work for themselves (or rather who cannot work within a system or for somebody else). This self-reliance extends to a resistance against asking for help and in letting somebody else help, comfort or reach them, so that they can often seem to be trouble free.

6. Insecurity

As a result of this self-reliance, the child learns vicariously rather than through trustworthy, intimate relationships. Instead of developing emotional intelligence, a sense of secure identity and worth, there will be an over-reliance on thinking things through. It is quite common that people who are ACoA can almost read a room before stepping into it as they have had to learn how to in order to survive. Rationalising emotions is a form of denial so that you appear to be feeling when actually you are repressing your feelings, and feelings have a nasty way of stewing, accruing and coming out sideways. The insecurity will feel bewildering to the person who has grown up in this environment as they have often convinced themselves of their own self-reliance and their lack of need so they will feel ashamed of the self-doubt. It will feel like a guilty secret, as if they are a fraud and it is very difficult to reassure them.

7. Guilty fury

The child will feel angry for the inconsistent behaviours and secrecy and for not being able to speak out for fear of causing more trouble. Often unconsciously, the child is angry with the parent for not having better self-esteem. How hard it is to love someone or to learn to love yourself if you come from someone who doesn't love themselves. But as the child can see the parent suffering, they will then feel guilty for feeling so angry and the anger turns inwards. Prone to outbursts of rage and then shame, the ACoA can be volatile; with no reliable guide to aid emotional regulation, they are at a high risk of addiction themselves as a means of coping.

How can you love another if you don't love yourself?

It seems cruel that one of our strongest influences in attraction should be the unresolved hurts and patterns of our pasts, so that we might recognise something difficult as familiar and translate it as attraction or love. Driven by our need to understand, we can therefore unwittingly seek out the very conflicts that hurt us in childhood. But so often all we do is repeat the same dynamic, but with different players, as we are the common denominator in all our relationships. I see it over and again: for example, if as a child you were the problem-solver, then problems are what you'll attract; if you are insecure and needy of attention, then it's an audience you will attract, not a partner; if you were neglected you are high risk of being drawn into a relationship where you feel invisible or taken for granted. Loving yourself can change all that as it means that you know that you matter, you feel kindly towards yourself and your behaviour reflects that truth. It becomes almost impossible to treat yourself badly and you transmit this into all your interactions with others, and attract the same. This isn't meant as permission to be self-indulgent or self-gratifying, but more to proactively acknowledge that you are just as valuable as everyone else. As I often say, you choose who you fall in love with, and if you want it to be a healthy, happy match, it must start with you.

The addict and the codependent relationship

The relationship characterised by a potent 'us against the world' dynamic is typical of the addict and the codependent interaction as it fulfils the need for intensity. It can feel like the best thing in the world to those two people when they connect; it can feel like true love, like they are now complete.

Thus the codependent is the perfect partner for the addict. Although, of course, they are an addict themselves, often the codependent will look 'normal'. The compulsive caretaker, whose role in life is to be the emotional shock absorber, the rock, the fixer of all ills, will fall in love with the charismatic but emotionally flawed addict.

Typically, the addict will begin to find the codependent controlling and suffocating and will start to pull away. Sensing this, the codependent will start to point out the faults in behaviour and try to pull the addict back into line, only causing more rebellion. The addict inevitably acts out and the codependent is offended, either engaging in argument or giving the cold shoulder – whatever it is, it is an intense response – until the addict complies, placates, and then the whole pattern can start again. This cyclical relationship pattern is intense and can include rows, affairs and violence. This is the relationship classroom for the children that follow.

. . . .

Jez and Harriet had been together since they were at school and when I met them, they were completely enmeshed emotionally. Working with them was difficult because they were so reactive to one another, to the slightest nuance, so there was little room between them for me to observe, challenge or disentangle. Often in relationships where one is the addict and the other the codependent, each also has characteristics of the other so that occasionally they swap roles. With Jez and Harriet this didn't happen and their roles as addict (liability) and codependent (caretaker) seemed set and well-defined. They came to me because they were worried about their daughter, who they felt was falling in with the wrong crowd. Listening to them, I heard a great deal of blame – Harriet 'had had enough' and Jez felt 'Harriet was driving everyone mad'. I found myself wondering what it was like to be their daughter, and agreed to work with them as a family.

. . . .

Apparently, the previous weekend had been a typical one. Harriet's parents were coming to lunch in an attempt to get the whole family together, and Jez and Harriet had agreed to go to a drinks party the night before 'just for one or two and to show our faces'. Harriet described how she had watched Jez from the other side of the room as he seemed to 'warm to his audience', clearly in the mood for a big night. She had gone over to him to remind him that they were only staying for a couple and he had dismissed her gregariously, suggesting she go home on her own, if she was tired. Humiliated, Harriet had waited a while, tried one more time to persuade him to join her and then had gone home on her own. All the while Harriet was speaking, Jez was trying to catch my eye as if to make a joke out of what Harriet was saying or to get me on side.

. . . .

Harriet described going into the house, incensed with rage and too agitated to go to bed until she heard Jez being dropped off around 4 a.m., at which point she had pretended to be asleep. Jez had stumbled in making some joke about Harriet being a party pooper and had gone off to sleep in the spare room. He woke the next day and his in-laws were already there. He had tried to pretend that he had overslept because of work but this time Harriet called him on it and he had felt ashamed, angry with Harriet for betraying him and for ruining the day. In the session, as Jez spoke, he was angry – all the while Harriet tried to engage me in eye contact as if to collude with me about how unreasonable Jez clearly was. It was crucial to notice they both had done the same thing, seeking to get me onside, and I wondered aloud if they did this with their children.

The roles we end up playing

Hero – Scapegoat – Lost Child – Mascot/Indulged (Wegscheider-Cruse, 1981)

The first child born into this environment has no peer; no equal to use as a sounding board to help understand the relational dynamic. Instead, they are the entire focus of this couple as a product of their union, as their child. But as the couple is so consumed with one another, this first child will always feel very alone or as if they are interrupting, which will go on to affect their own appetite in relation to intimacy. When the parents are connected and getting on well, this first child will feel so very special, affirmed and connected as the only representative of this intense, enmeshed union that looks like perfect love. But when it breaks down into resentment and blame, the loss is profound. To the first child, relationships feel unsafe.

. . . .

Sadie, Harriet and Jez's daughter, could remember when her mother would come home alone from an event and Sadie would call out for her. Harriet would come into her room, angry and impatient, asking, 'What do you want? Why aren't you asleep?' All Sadie remembers from those times was feeling 'wrong'.

. . . .

Hearing this in session, instead of responding to her daughter's experience, Harriet expressed feeling hurt. She felt she had been betrayed by her husband and also received no understanding from her daughter about how hard it had been for her (poor me). In the

*session, Sadie was able to express that this had left her feeling like
she did not matter and that she should have no needs.*

This feeling of being 'wrong' is one the hero child will seek to avoid by
aiming to be perfect, and in their achievement, they have no needs, so no
one can let them down. But this can leave the hero child isolated and fearful
of connection, no matter how successful they are otherwise. By default,
too, their success endorses the family system and allows the parents to
believe they are doing a good job. Until the second child comes along, as in
the case of Lexi, Jez and Harriet's 'problem child'.

. . . .

*Lexi was the child that had caused the parents to seek help. She
was taking drugs and they felt she was losing her grasp on her life.
Lexi was a force to be reckoned with and when she stepped into
my consulting rooms, I could feel the energy she brought. Sulking,
distrustful and angry, she provoked me to reject her as if rejection
was inevitable. She was jealous and angry towards her older sister,
Sadie, and protective of the next one down. Labelled 'difficult from
the start', Lexi couldn't see the point of therapy, especially as I
was asking her to give up drugs and drinking, at least for a while,
until we could see what was going on. I was asking her to give up
the one thing that made her feel safe, crazy as it sounds, and she
wasn't prepared to do it.*

. . . .

*With both parents stuck in this toxic cycle, Lexi had turned
to Sadie as a quasi-parent figure and Sadie had responded
accordingly, instinctively not trusting her parents to do a good
enough job, and so caretaking by parenting instead for them. Not
wanting to contribute to the family tension, Sadie started to deny
her own needs in favour of propping up the family by being the
good girl.* **Hero child – activated**

. . . .

*The destructive power struggle then evolved between Sadie
and Lexi, as Lexi's resentment grew against Sadie for not only
blocking Lexi from her parents, but also for being so perfect. Lexi's
behaviour became increasingly negative (as if filling the gap Sadie
left by being so good), disruptive and attention-seeking. Lexi
looked like the problem. Warming to this identity, Lexi began to
behave, say and even believe herself when she stated that she truly
didn't care about what other people thought.* **Scapegoat child –
activated.**

. . . .

*It wasn't until I managed to work with the parents so that they
began to change that Lexi became interested in working with me.
Then I began to hear why she wanted to take drugs and the painful
truths she was seeking to repress. The truth that she felt her
parents couldn't handle her. That she was too much for them. That
they didn't love her as they were so keen to blame her for their own
shortcomings. For her lack of faith in herself and, worst of all, her
lack of faith and respect for her parents.*

Any child following Lexi would have little time and space as Lexi made so
much 'noise' in her demands and acting out behaviours. Often this third
child will be quiet and just get on with their lives, neither good nor bad,
but not wanting or needing anything. Their invisibility allows the family to
believe that like the hero child, the third child is OK, again confirming the
problem as the scapegoat.

The lost child: Lexi's younger sister, Hannah, was sixteen years old when
I met her and it was as if she had no voice of her own: she was truly 'lost'.
The work needed was relational to give her time and attention because
she felt, at a constitutional level, that she was not entitled to either. The
therapist I referred her to worked with her for almost three years. In this
time, Hannah's patterns of seeking friendships with troubled people was

challenged and her own ability as an artist began to be recognised so that she followed through to pursue this as a career.

Mascot: Had there been another child, he or she would have been at risk of falling into the mascot or indulged role, making the family laugh, alleviating tension and attracting adoration. The apparent popularity can attract envy from the rest of the siblings and the indulgence means there is often no sense of what is enough, inspiring a shame-based sense of being too much. The downside is a deep-seated feeling that you are not as funny or talented as everyone made out, which can translate as an insecurity that is attention-seeking in its insatiable craving for external affirmation.

Thus the roles in brief are as follows and can explain the question many parents ruminate when they believe that they have treated each of their children the same, somehow ignoring any individual differences such as birth order or family circumstances. Understanding these details is not to attribute blame, but rather to find a way to gain purchase on slippery behaviours so as a parent you can feel proactive in your approach to prevention.

- **Hero:** good and perfect, with a fear of failing that motivates overt control. Self-reliant, they deny a need for help and instead offer advice and help as if a parent. The family feels they are not so bad because this person is so good. Prone to workaholism, alcoholism (but rarely out of control until middle age) and physical illness as a result of internalising the feelings.
  Needs: to allow an authority figure in, to receive comfort or help and to accept their human vulnerability so they can connect as an equal.

- **Scapegoat:** 'bad', angry, impulsive, the black sheep who feels rejected and full of shame so sets everyone up to confirm this rejection. As they adopt this role, everyone else can be good enough and blame them as the problem. Prone to addiction. Often the one most likely to see the truth in the family.

Needs: to become sober, acceptance that they are good enough, calm environment to soothe the hyper-alert defence mechanisms, curiosity in ability to see the truth.

- **Lost child:** ignored, quiet, invisible, with few conscious emotions though often anxious. Can be talented in music or art, as if seeking another form of communication. Often a good listener, and prone to falling into friendships with troubled people.
  Needs: to be seen and valued, and encouraged to pursue own thoughts and dreams.

- **Mascot:** entertaining and funny, the mascot child knows how to draw the fire, hiding pain with humour, while feeling like a fraud or inadequate. Avoidant and attention-seeking, they are often emotionally very immature.
  Needs: boundaries and to be taught what is enough, and self-esteem (as opposed to external affirmation as a way of feeling valuable); to grow up.

Nature or nurture

As soon as a baby is born, it's learning. Everything that happens, big or small, has an impact on how that baby's brain develops and, therefore, on how their personality develops, like sandpaper shaping a piece of wood. This is not only when you consciously approach your child to tell them something, but in your own behaviour and through the atmosphere of the family home. Thus, as parents, we are always teaching and we will all make some mistakes. The opportunity here is to be honest about that and sincere in your desire to make good. Most significantly for this chapter, consider how you teach your child how to have emotions. Whether to accept them (e.g. fear), whether to feel ashamed of them (e.g. anger), how to enjoy them (e.g. happiness and success) and how to go about expressing them (e.g. sadness). Simply, if a child has a parent who rages they will usually develop an all-or-nothing response to anger to cope, either by becoming very rageful themself or by withdrawing. Neither teaches a process of healthy anger and, worse, both can set up a foundation where there is a need to self-medicate: primed for addiction.

Often in my consulting rooms, a child or teenager will accuse a parent of being abusive or describe experiences the parent has never heard of before that have been traumatic for them. Over and again, the parents recoil in fear and shame of the judgement or consequences that might follow and naturally respond with denial, which only serves to frustrate their child, who then insists and maybe even embellishes the experience so that they feel heard. It's worth understanding what is understood as abuse so that you can listen to your child's experience with an open mind and begin to attend to the wounds, whatever they are, so that you and they can heal. I have provided a short guide below.

What is abuse?

Abuse is any violation of another person's rights. It can happen in extreme forms, which sadly we are increasingly familiar with hearing about and accept as abuse, such as actual physical or sexual violence against another person. But it can also happen in less obvious ways, such as through neglect, or when there is an abuse of power, like when a child is repeatedly shamed by the parent. Often I find there is resistance to using the term 'abuse' in these subtler forms because of its association with sexual abuse, for example. As if certain parental reactions are justified because of how badly the child has behaved. But my thought is that often the child has behaved in that way in the first place because of what they have experienced or witnessed.

Following are common forms of abuse that sadly can occur within the family home:

Physical – this includes any kind of physical behaviour that causes actual physical harm, including hitting, pushing, pinching, shaking, hair pulling.

Sexual – this is when someone is forced or persuaded to take part in any sexual activity as a child, or as an adult where they are resistant.

Emotional (or psychological) – repeatedly mistreating someone through, e.g. humiliation, intimidation, shaming, enmeshing, grooming, isolating or ignoring (bullying). For a child, even if they are not directly targeted, witnessing domestic abuse is a form of emotional and psychological abuse.

Neglect – this is as serious as any other form of abuse, whereby the person's needs are ignored and repeatedly overlooked.

Child abuse can be overt and aggressive in some way as above, or it can be as seemingly inconsequential as neglect: not giving the child enough healthcare, love and attention. But we now know that neglect is one of the most profound forms of abuse – it's hard to come back from being unseen and uncared for.

Sadly, if the parent is struggling in some way themself, without sufficient support or resources to cope, the fallout on the child is inevitable. This is not about blaming anyone; it's about spotting it and doing something about it as soon as you realise what's happening. If you are behaving towards your child in ways that you regret, and if you find yourself wanting to apologise, then take the risk to change and live the apology through your changed behaviour. Go to fellowship meetings, and work a recovery programme yourself. Show not only that you mean it, but also the invaluable lesson that change is possible.

Feeling traumatised

As a result of abuse, people become traumatised, and this can manifest in lots of ways that are extreme or again subtle, but which undermine the ability to have a happy, healthy, productive life. It's true that we reap what is sown.

- Difficulty with emotions and feelings and especially prone to anger, low mood or depression, anxiety and poor self-esteem.
- All-or-nothing responses so there is no grey area, only extremes (indulge/neglect, dominate/withdraw, confident/hopeless, love/hate).
- Disturbed sleeping and eating patterns, poor self-care (how hard it is to care about yourself without self-esteem).
- Distrust of anyone in power, which can manifest as avoidance or attacking and aggressive behaviour, even towards those who might want to help.
- Addiction problems.
- Suicidal and self-harming thoughts and behaviours.
- Intensity-seeking behaviours in terms of relationships, risk or physical danger.
- Poor physical health as the body and mind are closely connected and the body can present trauma in physical ways, such as extreme weight or auto-immune problems.
- Difficulty forming healthy relationships.
- Inappropriate loyalty to someone who treats them badly.
- Anti-social and criminal behavioural patterns.

So if your child is behaving in ways like those listed above, perhaps it's worth considering if they have been exposed to some form of abuse and if they might be traumatised in some way? Knowing what you are dealing with can help you to form a support plan that actually works. Eye Movement Desensitisation Therapy (EMDR) is an effective form of brief trauma therapy that works with the part of the brain responsible for survival and helps process partial memories or sensations so that the disturbed symptoms can recede.

Questions:
Are you an adult child of an addictive family system?
- Do you feel fear around people in positions of authority?
- Have you been a bully to avoid feeling bullied?

- Do you people-please and then feel lost and overlooked?
- Do you avoid people connecting with you through your self-reliance and disdain for others' input?
- Do you feel afraid of anger or criticism?
- Do you gravitate towards people who are big drinkers, drug takers or people who aren't really 'there' emotionally?
- Do you feel bad if you express your own needs and do you shame others for theirs?
- Are you so afraid of your own feelings that you make up how you feel instead?
- Are you so terrified of being left you stay in abusive relationships too long? Or perhaps you leave people as soon as they begin to care about you, abandoning first?
- Do people tell you that you are too hard on yourself, but you don't really know what they mean?
- Do you insist you come from a normal, happy family, even though deep down, when you think about where you find yourself today, this doesn't actually feel completely true?

Is my child growing up ACoA?
- Am I an addict or a codependent?
- Are they fearful of confrontation?
- Do they seek to caretake me or my partner?
- Do they show little respect for authority, or for me or my partner?
- Do they behave like a hero/scapegoat/lost child/mascot?
- If so, am I prepared to try and work on what they need instead of what they provoke in me?
- Does your child have the space, safety and opportunity to express how they feel without recourse?
- Does your child have to keep secrets about the family?
- What can I do to begin to address this?

Remember this is not about blaming anyone, it's about making sure that we can be the parents we want to be. To do that we have to know what we are made of so that we can take responsibility for what we pass on before we tackle our own children's behaviour.

Action suggestions if you are ACoA:

- Attend the ACoA fellowship (see The Essentials on page 221).
- Find a photo of yourself aged six to eight years, one that makes you feel affection. Talk to this part of yourself kindly and with interest, twice a day. Ask that child how they feel and what they want from you, the adult, today, and at the end of the day comment on how you fared. Getting well from ACoA starts when you begin to connect with the small child that was so hurt, and you learn to take proper care of him or her so that the experience of your childhood does not dictate how you behave as an adult or as a parent. Let the buck stop here.

7

SELF-ESTEEM

How I feel about myself drives who and what I attract into my life

When I think about the one thing that we could hone in on as the most important preventative measure for addiction, I would use those two little words 'self-esteem', i.e. how I feel about myself and therefore how I treat myself and others. As a parent, my level of self-esteem has a profound influence on that of my child. To be effective in parenting against addiction I must have good self-esteem.

What is self-esteem?

This is entirely about how you feel about you. Do you like you? Do you love you? Are you your best friend? Do you believe in yourself? Do you take proper care of yourself as a priority? If the answer to these questions is 'yes' then it is very unlikely that you will be able to put yourself through any experience that causes you unnecessary hurt or harm, because you care about yourself and your relationship with yourself is kind. Would you answer the same for your child?

If your child does not feel kindly towards themselves, they will be exposed to the worst critic on the planet. The hidden voice that can see all their shortcomings. The hidden voice that lacks so profoundly in self-esteem that it compares feelings against how everybody else looks so that every time it comes off worse. The lack of self-esteem that says there's something wrong with me, hide it, change it.

A lack of self-esteem (i.e. self-loathing) is the single most influential factor in a person's right to treat themselves badly. Self-esteem is therefore the best antidote. But you cannot force it or give it to someone – in fact, trying to can come across as shaming and confirm the lack of it! As a parent, you can only model it with humility, support it in your child though nurture and be patient as it grows through experience.

Self-esteem is saying 'I matter', and believing it. I don't matter more than you or less than you; I just matter, too. It is about accepting that I am flawed and being as interested in those flaws as I am in my skill set. It's about accepting that I am good at some things and I'm allowed to succeed. It's about being curious about myself, about what I feel and what I do. It's about being kind to myself so that I can grow and learn. It's about taking care of my basic needs because I deserve that attention. It's about feeling good enough in my own skin so that I have time, space and capacity to be interested and generous in the world.

As a parent, if I want these things for my child, I must risk attempting to learn them for myself first, so I can show the way.

Is it the same as confidence?

It is easy to say self-confidence is the same as self-esteem. It can look like you believe that you matter if you are prepared to stand up and be counted, put yourself forward, speak up for yourself and be seen. But interestingly for some, standing up and being confident can be an effective hiding place for poor self-esteem, as they hide in the distraction of performance. Often when I've worked with people in the world of celebrity, it is quite common to discover a façade under which a much more fragile, insecure persona exists. Perhaps the world of celebrity attracts exactly these kinds of people who seek affirmation from others as a way of shoring up their own sense of worth. But this then creates a dependence as without that platform the person might feel worthless. This is just as common in school with the class clown or at home with the one who plays the fool or shows off. Would it be such a huge leap to see the insecurity that craves the attention, that seeks to control what others think by making so much noise?

Unless you feel you matter irrespective of circumstance, just because you are a person, then it is hard to receive anything else that is good as you have no landing strip to receive on, no foundation on which to build.

It takes patience and calm to see through the façade and not be drawn to react, so that instead of being controlled by your child's provocation, you think for yourself. The work is all upfront and, as a parent, this can feel like too much effort is needed, especially if you work full-time or are tired. But if you do this from the outset, it will make it easier for you in the long term, as you stay connected to your child and you will not be distracted by their defences – and they will know it.

Having somebody feel good about themselves without being boastful or narcissistic is the key to the most profound method of prevention from addiction, a careful line to teach our children.

Why is self-esteem important?

An absence of self-esteem is likely to translate into a range of all-or-nothing behaviours because the baseline regulator, my relationship with myself, is damaged or compromised. Without a sense of worth irrespective of what I do or don't do, without an investment in myself as potentially useful or interesting in the world, without a sense of care about myself, I am unlikely to take proper care of myself, may expose myself to dangerous or harmful situations and at the very least feel lost. When I'm lost, I am vulnerable to being found by an influence I cannot measure, as all I am looking for now is certainty, identity, to satisfy or reassure my core social motive of belonging. In my addiction, I will find that certainty through substances, intense relation-ships and dramatic behaviours. For a while, it might feel like an answer, but for that while a lot of damage can be done. It's a chicken and egg situation: which comes first, the low self-esteem that causes me to act out through addiction, or does the acting out erode my self-esteem? The answer is both.

As a parent you need to be aware of your own experience of self-esteem, so you can see the part you are playing in your relationship with your child and adjust it to stay connected and accessible. But keep an eye on your child too and how they seem to feel about themselves by how they behave. It's an early sign that you might want to act on.

Self-esteem and vulnerability

If I believe that there is something wrong with me, and that deep down if you really knew me you wouldn't like me, then I will never show you who I actually am. I will never be vulnerable with you. Instead, I create other versions of myself in the hope that you might like them and that they might fit, like someone who is daring and devil-may-care, or someone who is a caretaker and a people-pleaser, always there for you. The tricky thing is that whatever version somebody puts up as a façade, no matter how popular they become as a result, they will not gain self-esteem from this. Conversely, what happens is a reinforced sense that the real me doesn't have a place in the world and the false me (which is preferred) is a lie, intensifying the feeling of being a fraud.

A child will be watchful of you as their parent and vulnerable to what you think, even if it doesn't seem that way. They will want to respect you and for you to be proud of them, in turn, so your pride has value, and if this doesn't happen, it hurts. As their parent, they will need you to be able to see them for what and who they are, and accept them. I've met many teenagers who cringe when their parents tell them how wonderful they are as they say that it's not realistic feedback, and some retort that it's all about the parents' wish for success or validation. Just as frequently, the teenager will be angry at criticism, exasperated by what they see as their parents' hypocrisy. To remain vulnerable in your company, a child needs to be able to show themselves and know you are there, truthful about who you are, trusting them to work it out for themselves. If they need help (and they trust you), they will ask. If they don't, think hard about why.

How do we teach or encourage self-esteem?

So often I meet parents who are frustrated in their attempts to teach their children self-esteem, describing how their child becomes withdrawn, defensive or irritated whenever they try to give them a compliment or affirm them in some way.

The first step in promoting self-esteem in another is to consider your presence as the messenger. Do your words hold weight? Are you teaching 'do as I say, not as I do', or do you practise what you preach? In other words, will your child want what you've got, because if they don't, they are less likely to do what you suggest. Sometimes the feeling of offence a parent feels when their child won't be reassured by them is a truthful indicator of where a part of the problem lies. Developing your own core of self-esteem is a powerful step towards promoting the same in your child.

. . . .

Gemma was twenty-two and I had worked with her so that she was in early recovery from anorexia and self-harm. In session with her mother, she said the words: 'I can't take from you even though I want to as you haven't got anything to give.' Her mother was always busy, very practical, never seemed to pay much atten-tion to how she felt or needed emotionally. Her daughter's illness had terrified and infuriated her as she was a problem-solver and it had been beyond her power to fix. This in itself was interesting information and led me to think about why her daughter had 'chosen' this form of addiction, so out of her mother's reach: what was she trying to prompt or say. It seemed to me that if her mother learned how to care about herself, and brought that 'language' into the relationship with her daughter, it might help. It transpired that her mother, a successful businesswoman, was the hero child of an alcoholic father and emotionally cold mother and her safe place was to fix problems and be OK. Working through this history allowed her to begin to open up channels of interaction with her daughter that were intimate and meaningful

and which they later revealed had transformed their relationhip
beyond recognition.

The first step in dealing with your child's self-esteem is to make sure you are in good relationship with yourself, so that you're showing as well as telling. From this position, it's important to be able to properly hear what your child is saying in their poor self-esteem. Maybe like the mum of seemingly confident Keira in the last chapter, your child is telling you they have no friends or that they can't do something – whether you agree or not, it's important to actually hear where they are coming from. Too often parents will react by telling their child that what they are saying or experiencing isn't true, which will only serve to drive their thinking underground. 'He who is convinced against his will is of the same option still.' As with Keira's mother, hear what your child is saying and repeat it. 'I hear you think you have no friends' – and then comment on how that sounds to you – 'that sounds really painful.' You don't have to agree, but you do have to hear. So you can say 'it's not how I see it, but I am not you, so I guess we have different viewpoints on this'. Leave your perspective there as a valid alternative, but try not to use it to counter their view.

If you don't trust your child to come up with their own solutions, then you will seek to give them answers yourself. Remember, rescue creates a victim. In giving your child the answer, you confirm that you don't believe they will come up with it themselves. Ask your child what they want to do about it, what thoughts they have – brainstorm, including the funny ideas, and ask if you can keep talking about it and see how it goes. Let them know you're there to help by listening or commenting. They will face many problems in life and always seeking an answer might suggest that there is a life to be had that is without problems!

If you struggle with this, it may be because you struggle with seeing your child struggle and if that's the case I would suggest you take this seriously enough to work it through. Whether on your own or with a therapist, try to think about why you cannot tolerate witnessing someone struggle. Understanding what happened to you will help you to understand why you cannot tolerate witnessing your child's difficulties, and separate their process from your own, so that you become more resilient and tolerant of your child's growing up process and more useful to them as a result. Struggling can be a good thing. It can be a way to develop strength and personal perspective in relation to friends, peers and environment and is a lot better than not struggling or giving up. Pain can be a great teacher as long as it is properly managed or contained.

Self-esteem and mental health – where it can go wrong

In the event of a crisis or problem of some kind, where a child has learned that help helps, they're more likely to ask for it. Through this process the child learns not only that they don't have to do things on their own, but each time, they learn another way of addressing a problem. This helps them to develop and grow into a resourced and confident person, who is increasingly resilient, with the humility to work with others.

However, where experience has taught a child that they will be hurt or shamed if they ask for help, or that it's not OK for them to struggle then they will panic when a crisis or problem presents itself. In their fear and distrust, they will probably get defensive and seek to blame or avoid what is actually going on and sometimes divert their attention to a maladaptive behaviour such as self-harm or drinking or even just through creating drama. This means that they avoid the simple learning process of going through something difficult and generate all sorts of other difficulties that not only distract their attention but may overwhelm. All the child learns in this process is that problems cause more problems and so are to be avoided and as a result of this cyclical negative reinforcement, their self-esteem goes down.

I believe what I was taught by my friend and mentor Anthony McLellan, that emotions are what we have the most of and know the least about; handle them or they will handle you. If your child is upset, it doesn't justify you getting upset as well. Instead, it requires you to stop and listen, to show them it's safe for them to do the same, and so you have a firm starting place from where to work things out. Sometimes it means you have to learn to help your child to breathe deeply so that they learn to pause and so that feelings don't dictate their behaviour (see page 11, breathing exercise). This is where self-esteem can begin as they face their fears and yet still do the next right thing. This kind of manual override allows someone to have feelings but to be so much more – 'I am not my feelings!'

Practice makes perfect, and the more you are able to encourage your child to attempt things that might be difficult the better as long as success is measured as much in terms of learning and attitude as in outcome. If your child approaches a challenge in their self-esteem, they can learn without feeling shamed, try without feeling stupid, want without feeling needy and ask without feeling a burden – because they accept they are 'only' human and no better and no worse than anyone else, just themselves. This can start in their relationship with you.

Actions:

Help your child to find their voice: this can be through singing or dancing, or maybe a walk in the middle of nowhere where they can make a big noise and take up some space, jumping, shouting, so that they get a sense of their size and capacity. If you're able to suggest this, then encourage their thoughts about what it would be like for them to manage their unique energy to their best advantage.

For you (and once you've mastered it you can pass it on to your child but do it yourself first so you understand it):
- Remove yourself from any triggering scenarios so you can reflect on what was triggering about them – remember triggering means you are responding to what's happening now but fuelled by something in your past – that bit is your responsibility to deactivate.
- Don't suppress your feelings: sharing how you feel with someone you trust can help you feel a bit lighter.
- Don't react on your first thought, take time out before responding and be curious about what you think/feel.

- Say 'no' if you need to; say 'yes' if you know that you're avoiding something.
- Write down ten things *now* that you can do that are caring and estimable acts so you have them to prompt you when you're feeling low.
- Ask yourself what is preventing you from doing things that you want to do.
- Ask yourself if you use your strengths to feel better than others or if you can you simply enjoy them.
- Do your feelings dictate how you feel about yourself? And if they do, can you begin to change that and allow your emotions to be up and down, remaining curious in your ability to learn and grow?
- Is the way you feel about yourself your own point of view? Or have you taken on somebody else's?
- Do you actually respect that other person's point of view? Or are you just afraid of them?
- Start to look at who you are and bank the things you like about yourself.
- Make sure you get enough sleep, that you relax, connect, exercise, practise gratitude and manage your anger with curiosity.
- Now begin to teach this to your child!

8

GUILT, SHAME AND ANGER

Love doesn't hurt

The experience of guilt, shame and anger are vital in any human inter-action, but only if they are healthy and operating from an active foundation of love and respect. Unhealthy or toxic guilt / shame / anger can be three of the most destructive emotions to pollute any family dynamic. Accepting that these normal, human emotions exist in any household, but that there are constructive as well as destructive ways to experience them, puts you in the driving seat to be proactive in how they influence your family. Each has value in terms of shaping your child to be responsible, in terms of how they represent themselves and in their right to personal happiness.

Guilt

The feeling of guilt reflects the relationship between your internal moral code and the world, between how you want to be or who you think you should be and how and who you actually are. It tells you when you (feel like you) have overstepped the mark, whether that's in something you've done or said, or even felt. It's like an internal alarm system that makes you aware that you are compromising something you value.

In almost all my interactions with parents, at least one of each has spent sleepless nights combing through their child's history from birth, noting every single thing they feel they have done wrong and that might have

contributed to that child's problems. The guilt they report can be debili-
tating as there is no going back or rewriting history. What's done is done.
I appreciate their honest report because it gives me the information I need
to understand not just about what did or didn't happen, but in relation to
how the family values have been compromised, which tells me about the
culture of the family. Often parents speak about how they have sought to
discipline their child and feel guilty for losing their temper, while in the
same sentence ameliorating that guilt by justifying it against the child's
behaviour, as if the child is responsible for what the adult did. This place
of internal conflict has no resolution as they go round and round in this
eternal argument. The real value of the guilt is that it serves as a signpost
to what needs to change.

The danger of parental guilt

There is a downside to this kind of forensic soul-searching that would place
the parent or parents at the centre of their child's demise. In believing
yourself to be the problem, or the cause, three significant things occur:

1. As the only cause, you are by default the 'only' solution, and
   this is an issue of control.
2. In owning that you are the cause, the other party – in this case
   the child – can abdicate all responsibility as everybody knows it
   is or was your fault.
3. When one parent decides that it's all their fault, usually the
   other parent is driven to counterbalance this view by seeking to
   make the child equally responsible.

None of these options is productive in terms of resolving any current issue.

How to intervene

It is only when the parent is able to be honest that a healthy and constructive communication about the past can happen between parent and child. When the guilt still exists the child can abdicate responsibility as 'everyone knows it's mum's/dad's fault', commensurately serving the parents with a 'mortal blow' of blame, a power no child should have. None of us is perfect, so why promote it as a goal? It is unlikely to motivate and instead sets an unachievable bar so that the child may feel a failure no matter the achievement (and of course, the parent setting that bar is probably just as hard on themselves, even if they seek to hide it).

Actions:

- Go through your history – note down the events you feel guilty about as a parent (you will probably have been torturing yourself with this anyway, so let's get it down!).
- Underline what you feel has contributed to the issues you see in your child today.
- Ask yourself how you feel – notice if you use a feelings word (there is a list of the negative feelings many people struggle to identify at the end of this book) or a judgement such as fine/good/bad/OK.
- Notice your inner conflict as you slip into guilt and then get annoyed as you defend yourself – neither is helpful.
- Once you have noted the things you feel guilty for, write them out and see if you can establish a theme, such as over-giving so that you have kids who demand all the time and then you get annoyed and shout at them and then you feel guilty; or shaming your child for 'take, take, take', when perhaps it's you not being able to say 'no'.
- In what way has your behaviour contradicted your moral code (or so that you behave out of character in your view)? This is important in understanding why this happened, given how you wish you were or would prefer to be, and to explore whether your expectation of yourself is realistic – whether your moral

code is your own or someone else's imposed upon you and to be curious around your own responses and behaviour rather than judgemental.

- Within all this, you will begin to find that you can forgive yourself again and again without denying your part in the inter- action. But in that self-forgiveness you can become honest and therefore accountable to your child for whatever they would care to bring to your attention as, in their view, influential in their negative symptoms.

If a child feels guilt

Good!

It's important that a child feels guilt and shame as part of a healthy devel- opmental process, but it is equally important these feelings are constructive and allow development and growth rather than facilitate a collapse into poor self-esteem and self-loathing. Learning how to take responsibility is an important part of learning how to be socialised, and this will only happen if the experience of owning up and taking responsibility for something you regret is not too punishing. Thus when a child is found to be guilty of a particular behaviour, they must be held accountable so that they under- stand what they have done is not acceptable and be encouraged to consider why they did what they did and accept that there are other ways in which they could have dealt with it that might be more constructive.

Saying sorry and being sorry are two different things: one reflects words and the other a change in behaviour. Too often in my consulting room I have met with families who have lost faith in the word 'sorry'. Sometimes parents introduce consequences to reinforce a learning process, such as being grounded or the removal of technology. All I will say is that the punishment must meet the crime or the child will only learn that the parent is punitive or unreasonable and the consequence will not promote any productive link to help the child learn anything beyond developing ever better skills to obscure what they are doing.

The value of shame

Shame is an important emotion that allows us to feel embarrassed as we navigate the interpersonal boundary between how we feel and what we want or don't want in relationships and in the world. It allows us to be vulnerable and relational as we experience the intimacy of brushing up against other people's needs and wants and the systems and constructs that map out our environment. But when that embarrassment converts to feeling ashamed there is a danger of a person internalising that moment as a personal flaw or mistake which will go on to compromise their ability to repeat the experience and to learn in a constructive way.

Healthy vs toxic shame

Different to guilt, an uncomfortable feeling around something you said or have done that contradicts your value system, shame makes it personal so that it's not about what you've done or said, it's about you: you are what's wrong; you are the mistake and when shame takes hold in this way your self-loathing can take over, leaving the door wide open for self-destructive behaviours. Addiction is fuelled by a shame core that means it is possible for a person to wilfully behave in ways they know are self-harming and futile.

When we feel unbearable shame, the response can be violence, drug abuse and other forms of self-harm. We feel the shame of our bodies, so we harm ourselves by cutting or burning; we feel the shame of our appetite and presence, and so we harm ourselves through eating disorders; we feel ashamed of our worth, and so become codependent or a workaholic in an effort to prove ourselves by doing more than anyone else to feel the same as anyone else. The prevalence of these patterns among many more in our society indicates that something is profoundly wrong, and it's replicated in families where the message from parent to child is, 'if you don't do as I say then there is something wrong with you'. The threat that follows is rejection and abandonment through disapproval. This kind of relational experience with a parent can set the attachment template at 'insecure'. It is vital when we seek to criticise, instruct or discipline that it is the behaviour we are seeking to adjust, not the child themselves – don't make it personal!

．．．．．．．．．．．．．．．．．．．．．．．．．．．．．．．．．．．．．．

Cole was so riddled with shame that he simply couldn't be honest and so was profoundly isolated. All he sought to do in session with me was to position himself in line with what he thought I wanted from him. When he realised he couldn't please me, Cole would become frustrated and angry, moving between blaming me for not doing my job properly and blaming the people in his life for setting him up to be this way, so that he was always so profoundly misunderstood, then each and every time shaming himself as useless, hopeless, disappearing into a depressive state of 'what's the point'. This man had a significant history of childhood abuse, which he had never spoken about, believing much of it to have been his fault as he hadn't stood up to his abuser. The most intense abuse happened between seven and nine, when Cole had been subjected to repeated verbal and sometimes violent physical behaviour. In order to control the profound fear, pain and isolation that he had felt at the time, he had blamed himself and then gone on to repeat this in all his adult relationships so that he (unconsciously) invited people to confirm his core belief of being worthless so that they also abused or rejected him. This is the power of shame. Recovery is a long, slow process of encouraging the individual to step away from the security of being at the bottom of the pile with nowhere to fall, so they begin to believe that they actually matter. As in Cole's case, this can be incredibly painful as they anticipate rejection in every interaction.

The work as a therapist, and therefore perhaps the parallel preventative work as a parent, is to acknowledge that that is how a child might view the world so that, as in Cole's case, they think they know what I am thinking and try to force me to deliver accordingly. I need to be sufficiently secure in my own skin as a therapist, or as a parent, to respond with my own reality and for that to be sincere and consistent.

Whenever I speak about shame to clients and their families it often serves to confuse and then suddenly the simple message comes through. Shame as a way for someone to blame themselves so that no one else can blame them without them getting there first. A provocative victim, the person will set you up to reject them and you won't see it coming. Like sailing into the Bermuda Triangle, around your shame-based child you lose yourself so that the feeling of content you had disappears, and you find yourself shouting horrible things at your child. As a parent, you need to know how to navigate toxic shame so that you do not fuel it, inadvertently or otherwise, as it can be infuriating to be around and terrifying when you fall into its trap and feel like you're part of the problem.

Shaming your child

Sadly, it is all too common for a parent to shame their child, albeit often out of fear or ignorance. I don't only hear about it in my consulting rooms where at least I have an opportunity to intervene, I see it in the supermarket, walking down the street, it's all too commonplace, painful to witness and the consequences are profound. The sorts of interactions I'm talking about are when there is a distortion of the power dynamic between parent and child and the parent is telling the child negative things about themselves: that they are difficult/a little s***/lazy/nasty/greedy . . . you get the picture. It may well be that the child is displaying behaviours that might warrant these descriptions, but that is very different to them actually being these things as part of their personality. The part that we as parents often forget is how powerful we actually are just by being the parents. That despite how we feel in that moment, which influences our reaction or a judgement, we have to remember how we want to communicate that to the child in the most constructive way. Offloading and shaming is unlikely to promote positive change and growth. Even adjusting the comment to 'I find you difficult' is very different to saying 'you are difficult' because it includes you, the parent, in the relationship interaction. It's your stuff too!

When a child is persistently shamed by a parent, they will lose self-esteem. This means they lose the ability to like themselves or to want to take care of themselves. In reaction to this, they will either go into what the therapy world refers to as feeling better than everyone else, or not good enough.

Better than

They will become arrogant, a narcissistic defence against feeling profoundly inadequate and terrified of being caught out as a fraud. This can make your child come across as aggressive, critical and scorning and it may feel threatening being close to them as you are drawn into a pattern of stroking and enabling the outer façade while feeling ever more distant.

Not good enough

To see themselves as hopeless is safer, as then they have nowhere to fall in anyone's estimation, and so your child will begin to lose the ability to ask for anything, to put themselves forward for anything and gradually lose 'their voice' in the world. They will be prone to attaching to someone who seems certain (controlling) as if abdicating responsibility for themselves entirely, such is their worthlessness.

In both cases, they will be angry inside even if they don't show it, or sometimes even know it themselves – whether that is overt aggression or passive aggression, they are angry because whether they are conscious of it or not it is a defence and not the 'true' them. So they will be prone to picking fights or self-harming from a state of isolation. They will be prone to what might appear to be random or unreasonable acts of violence on themselves and at times on others.

Witnessing your child decline into this kind of behaviour is excruciatingly painful. It will leave you feeling useless and completely unable to do anything about it, as a parent you stand by helplessly. My advice to you is to take the time to regroup yourselves. See a therapist and take a look at yourself and the core components of the family home and give yourself an emotional MOT! This means you would consider your responses and expectations through the lens of your own childhood so you can see yourself as involved in your child's behaviour, but more importantly it gives you something you can do.

What is anger?

Anger is nature's primary resource for defence, an instinctive and necessary response to fear and pain and vital for a long and happy life, but it requires self-regulation as there is a dark side too. Uncontrolled or repressed anger will cause untold pain and damage in the form of resentment, born of unreasonable expectations, or rage, the feeling stored when we have been shamed.

Physical symptoms may include headache, tension in the body, held breath, clenched fists, grinding teeth, flushing (face and/or neck), sweating, paling ('white with anger'). Some people feel it like a slow burn rising up through them and others like a rush or a flood. Adrenaline and noradrenaline course through the blood propelling you into action in response to a flight, fight or freeze event. In the brain, the amygdala (responsible for emotion) is overstimulated and the frontal lobe (responsible for reasoning) is overwhelmed. Regularly being in this state can cause damage to the heart, liver, kidney, immune system and mood, often leading to anxiety and depression, and is considered a major player in ill health and premature death.

Healthy anger

It is of fundamental importance to teach your child a healthy relationship with anger and this will start with your own relationship with this primal emotion. How you react when you get angry is the first place your child learns about anger, whether that's about them or in relation to somebody else, they are watching and they are learning. One day it is likely that whatever you do will be thrown right back in your face so be ready. If you are the kind of person who feels victimised and complains from a 'poor me' perspective, it is likely in their teen years you will feel that your child is doing exactly that to you, treating you badly so you feel a victim. But perhaps what they might (unconsciously) be doing is asking you to work through the position you have taken so that you are no longer available to be victimised?

As importantly, your reaction to your child's anger is a significant influence on how this emotion develops in them and in the environment at home. Anger is an assertion of human right and self-respect and must be encouraged but contained. You do not want your child to grow up in the world without healthy anger in their repertoire as without it you set them up to be without the right of self-defence, which leaves them wide open to being exploited and taken for granted. This means that home is the teaching ground for this challenging emotion. It doesn't mean that, open arms, you encourage anger, but it does mean that when your child starts to get angry you listen, you acknowledge the emotion, affirm the point without necessarily agreeing, and you teach them how to stay within manageable limits so that their anger does not dominate or threaten. If, for any reason, you are afraid of conflict or of anger this will be extremely difficult for you to do and therefore my recommendation would be for you to sort out your own relationship with anger, possibly with a therapist, before taking this on.

Expectation, resentment and the Drama Triangle

Fed by thwarted expectation, resentment is present in almost every relapse, which makes it one of the most important of The Core Characteristics™ to address and to devise coping strategies around it as a way of prevention. Resentment is played out in the Drama Triangle, which is fundamentally a relational dynamic of 'poor me/bad you; poor you/bad me'. Circulating around blame and shame, in either of these places a person can abdicate responsibility, abandon self-esteem and indulge themselves in self-destructive behaviours, as a way of coping with a relationship or an interaction. Later in this chapter, I will introduce a mechanism to step out of this Drama Triangle, but in brief, the way to avoid it is to develop curiosity as an antidote to offence.

Instead of moving into resentment, I suggest a heightened awareness of disappointment as the early warning that one of your expectations has been triggered so that when you feel disappointed you refer inwardly to whatever wishful thinking (often in the form of 'should' or 'if only') that has been thwarted. This could be something as seemingly petty as feeling enraged that your child doesn't come when you call for supper or that they don't listen to you, or when you ask them to calm down they ignore you, so you get furious. The 'should' or 'if only' relating to your expectation that your child respond to you in a certain way can create real problems in a family dynamic as it perpetuates a good guy/bad guy identity that's hard to shake. Perhaps your child feels the same about you, too. What's important is to challenge your immediate reaction of offence and become curious as to why you have got so upset instead of blaming your child (or parent) for how you feel.

Many parents might dismiss what I am suggesting here in the simple belief the child should respect a parent, simply because they are the parent, and I absolutely challenge this. If that parent does not have self-respect then it is very unlikely that the child will respect them.

The Five Things™

I developed this technique over fifteen years ago and always thought I'd come up with a better name! But the five things it was and so it remains: five things to do or say to get yourself out of an interaction that is charged with blame and shame. The key is that the outcome isn't to win anyone over or control anyone else, it's to represent yourself with dignity and respect.

So often when I work with parents they tell me that their child can 'press their buttons' and of course (to many parents' disappointment, as their expectation is that I will provide answers to better control the child) the answer is that they need to deactivate their own buttons first! It's not about controlling the child . . . yet. The first crucial step is to regain a position of respect yourself.

I often use the Drama Triangle as a way to illustrate the kinds of conflicts that my clients need to learn to better navigate. Central to the thinking in Transactional Analysis, Karpman's Drama Triangle (see diagram below) offers three positions in an interaction of conflict that circulates around blame and shame (self-blame): the persecutor – accusing and self-righteous, confident to point out who and what is in the wrong; the victim – hopeless, helpless, worthless, what's the point; the rescuer – fixing, resolving, the intermediary.

People often recognise themselves in one or more of the roles so that they often feel like a victim (poor me) or compelled to rescue (because the victim needs me or the persecutor is out of order and I'm the one to step in), but the roles are interchangeable and if you are one, you are all three.

The interactions circulate around attribution of blame and shame (remember that shame is blame turned inwards). It is an intense way of interacting as someone is always to blame and there is always a drama to deal with. Somebody's head must always roll, so it can also generate a deep impulse to avoid blame at any cost.

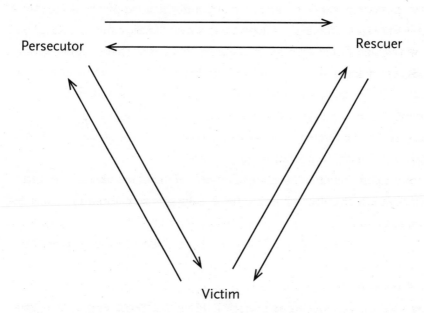

'The Drama Triangle' by Dr Stephen B. Karpman, www.karpmandramatriangle.com

Blame, fear of blame = defensive adult (shame)

In a family where there has been a lot of blaming, where whoever gets the blame carries the weight of responsibility of fault, the children are likely to grow up to be avoidant of taking responsibility and to be extremely defensive of taking the blame. This can manifest in a variety of ways such as in self-righteous behaviour, always being right or fine, never having issues, never needing help or conversely at the other end of the scale so profoundly affected that they cannot be blamed lest it hurt them too much or tip them over the edge into despair (shame). This all-or-nothing behaviour is symptomatic of an avoidance of the intimacy of relationship within which, as we have already established, there must be the experience of healthy shame or guilt as a result of human vulnerability interacting. At the merest hint of blame or of something going wrong that person will become powerfully triggered, even in adulthood, decades after the childhood environment is relegated to history, that they become so defensive alienating the very people who are closest to them.

If you recognise this dynamic is playing out, then you are lucky because you're one step towards resolving it. Most of the time, when I do the work with the Drama Triangle, people start by recognising themselves in one role or another, then they graduate to recognise the other common players in that triangle with them. In a matter of weeks, they will usually begin to see the Drama Triangle playing out 'everywhere'. Avoiding the Drama Triangle is hard, as for a moment it feels good because of the certainty it delivers. On the Drama Triangle, you know who are the good guys, the bad guys: you know where you stand. In exploring your expectations, there is no immediate relief and sometimes it just seems fairer and right to blame. But if you think about where blame actually gets you, you may reconsider this point of view.

The Five Things™

Essential to the effectiveness of this simple technique is a goal of self-representation with dignity and respect, being clear about your perspective and grateful to have some appreciation of the other person's point of view. This is not about changing anyone, it's about communicating and being curious. If you try to use The Five Things™ as a way to control an outcome, you are back on the Drama Triangle – blaming and shaming.

1. **Gratitude** – people often ask me what they're supposed to be grateful for if, for example, they are being shouted at. The answer is to at least be grateful you have realised you are on the Drama Triangle and that you have an opportunity to change your behaviour.

2. **Repeat verbatim** as much as possible of what the other person has said. This is important to show that you were listening. Most people say, 'I hear you', which is almost inevitably followed by the word 'but', indicating that the words may have been heard but not the meaning. This will only serve to fuel frustration and conflict.

3. **Acknowledge** the wisdom of what the other person is saying. Stand in their shoes for a moment and try to understand, and genuinely appreciate where they are coming from. This doesn't mean you are saying that they are right and you are wrong, what it is saying is that you genuinely have the confidence and capacity to take on another person's point of view, even when it appears to be in opposition to your own. This will help develop empathy and respect in your relationship.

4. **Offer your point of view**. It's important to notice the word 'offer'. This needs to be articulated with words like, 'may I tell you where I'm coming from?', as a contributory piece of information. If the other person doesn't want to hear where you're coming from, they won't listen anyway no matter how you put it so you are wasting your breath.

5. **Gratitude.** Thank you for listening.

This is how you step off the Drama Triangle. If you are wondering 'but that won't make my child do what I want them to do', you're right it may not in the short term. But in the parent–child relationship, we are looking at the long term and trying to promote a relationship of respect, and this comes as a result of patient, respectful interaction, starting with you!

Aggression vs assertiveness

A simple description would be to say that aggression might be to stand up *to* someone else while assertiveness is standing up *for* yourself. Aggression is seeking to control another person while assertiveness is seeking self-representation with self-control. There is very little justification in my view for aggression. Of course it happens, and as human beings we will all fall foul of indulging the self-righteous power that comes with the feeling of aggression. Rarely does it seem to bear positive consequences whereas assertiveness time and again brings results. You can feel the self-respect when someone is assertive in a proper way; standing up for themselves, representing themselves, but not trying to control anyone or anything – just being themselves. It's a very attractive quality. It's a chicken-and-egg situation whereby when somebody has a negative core belief, a shame-based view that they are worthless and will be rejected, then how often that becomes their reality. Equally somebody who believes they should be treated with respect often demands the same. It seems that how we feel about ourselves is an important indicator of how we will invite others to treat us, and that relationship with our self is predominantly shaped by our early childhood relationships and vicarious learning. You can help your child learn this vital difference by choosing not to exploit the power you have and being aggressive, but instead letting your child know you, and learn to respect how you handle conflict. I have met many teenagers who report feeling humiliated when their parent gets aggressive with someone else, a waiter or someone like that. They determine never to be like that and are more prone to the kind of passive aggression familiar in the repressed anger state.

Fault vs accountability

There is an important difference between blaming or feeling blamed and accepting and/or feeling accountable for something and that is self-esteem. The experience of feeling to blame is a shaming experience that means you personally are at fault, whereas recognising accountability allows a process of learning through taking responsibility for a behaviour or action. The latter encourages maturity, whereas the former will inhibit the maturation process, diverting instead into self-centredness.

Thus when you want to hold somebody accountable for something that they have done right or wrong, it is important that you point at the behaviour or the asset or defects of character rather than making it personal. This is done by quite literally saying, for example, 'you handled that really effectively' rather than 'you're brilliant at that'. It is also achieved by adding yourself into the dynamic so that the feedback is recognised as subjective, for example, 'I felt that you handled that really effectively'.

When you don't feel anger

When people are unable to express their anger directly, they can indirectly experience their angry feelings through others or as passive aggression so that they feel judged and guilty. An absence of anger is as significant as its overt presence. When anger is repressed, it's usually because the person believes that feeling to be 'unacceptable', usually because at an early age, they have learned to deny their own anger or their own emotional process, perhaps because they were hurt themselves or they bore witness to anger and hurt. Possibly associated with pain and shame, these people will often insist and resist 'going there'. (This is often a feature of codependency/ self-harm/eating disorders.) As a result, there may be consequences such as stress, depression or an impact on the immune system. Someone who represses their anger may project it onto other people too, so that they see anger in others while denying it in themselves or they may be critical or sarcastic, obscuring their anger in humour. When a parent denies their anger, their child is an obvious conduit instead so that they may appear disruptive, but it's the parent's anger they are displaying. It's therefore important to look out for how each member of the family experiences anger and for it to be visible. If you can't see it, it's a problem!

Control through threat

When control takes the form of threat, some children react by provoking it as if to control when the threat is realised, as we have discussed in previous chapters, accepting that the attack is inevitable. But if the children themselves are threatening a rageful outburst followed by brooding shame, the family will often seek to counter control as they tread on eggshells, trying to position or manipulate them so that they don't erupt or fall apart. This can often create the very conflict they wanted to avoid as it reinforces the feelings of shame the child inevitably feels as if they are being treated like they are a monster. The lack of trust in either party to be able to hold a respectful, calm position means that everybody starts to deploy tactics to control the environment. Often the most controlling people are those who have experienced profound fear very young.

Actions:
Ten ways to help your child better manage their angry feelings:
1. Help them get interested in their own emotional process.
2. Understand if it's fear that is motivating the anger.
3. Encourage 'I' statements instead of 'you' accusations.
4. Encourage 'won't' over 'cant' or 'want to' over 'have to'.
5. Notice the impact of anger on breathing and body and teach them to take charge of those reactions by relaxing and breathing before they express themselves, including posture and eye contact.
6. Help them to count to ten before expressing themselves. You are not encouraging an avoidance of the anger, you're encouraging a respectful expression of the same.

7. Journalling is a really good tool to use as a decompression tank which allows someone to sift their feelings from the facts.

8. Help your child to notice if they're taking everything personally and to ask themselves if this is really about them.

9. Help your child see what stresses them and to deal with that conflict while showing them that they can express themselves and be angry and still be loved.

   Sincerely apologise if you need to and try to accept their apology if they genuinely give it.

10. Most importantly let your child know you are not afraid of their anger, and that you can help them to learn how to experience anger in a healthy and productive way. (If you don't feel able to, then take the time to work with a therapist so that you can overcome your own experience of fear that prejudices your ability to contain as a parent.)

Rage

Archived anger, old and misfiled so it sits there like a bomb, liable to go off under stress, a misplaced comment or event, or due to tiredness or guilt. Rage is fuelled by 'yesterday's news' and has no place in a healthy person's 'today'. Rage attacks are emotional purges, where old emotion is taken out on another person. These are often followed by denial and shame. The person who suffers from rage has usually been badly hurt in the past and has hidden it, even from themselves. They are often the hardest to reach, as they often do not believe that their behaviour is as bad as it is. They are also difficult to be around as they offload onto others, who are then hurt by the outburst.

Regret

Many parents I meet are riddled with regret as they judge themselves harshly, wishful that they could go back and change the past. Instead, they compensate in the present day by indulging otherwise unacceptable behaviour, or by having 'soft' boundaries that reflect their conflicted self-esteem, making them targets for disrespect. As their children continue to act out, the parents continue to blame themselves, regretting past 'mistakes', like wishing that they hadn't punished in that way, changed schools, moved house, had to work, had intervened when they didn't, that they had divorced, had said no when they said yes or vice versa. But regret, like guilt, is only valuable as a signpost to what needs changing today. Living in the past only perpetuates the pain and enables more disrespectful behaviour. We are all human.

Questions:
- Do you feel unhealthy shame (often embarrassed or feeling humiliated)?
- Do you know where this comes from? Is it old triggers playing out today?
- Write these down so you know they are old and not current and have no place in your world today!
- How do you behave when you feel this kind of shame?
- How would you like to behave – can you fake it to make it?!
- What gets in the way?
- Can you identify moments in the last week where you have felt healthy anger, resentment and rage – can you write down an example of each?
- What's the difference between each?
- How can you stop blaming and start to see the part you play in your own angry experience?
- What are you teaching?

9

MODELLED BEHAVIOUR

We teach best what we most need to learn

We are none of us perfect and modelled behaviour has a huge impact on how a message from parent to child is delivered. So, as parents, we are always teaching, and a good enough goal is to be 'a good enough mother'. For those who are interested, the term 'good enough parent' was first coined by D.W. Winnicott (Winnicott, 1953), reflecting a healthy diversion from the concept that there is such a thing as the perfect parent. I, like many others in my field, support this concept.

The simple message of this chapter is that *you matter*!

Whenever I say that to a parent in my consulting room or at a school, the immediate response is to nod and agree, swiftly followed by 'yes, but . . .'. There's nothing more normal than the parental desire to secure your child before attending to your own needs, prioritising all resources towards your children. But what's important to understand is that how you treat yourself is a massive and often overlooked influence on you and how your child learns to do the same.

Most parents that I meet feel deskilled around their children, sometimes afraid of them and thus walking on eggshells; other times, the parent expresses that they don't know their child anymore or that although they love them, they don't like their child anymore. Although addiction is not the only reason for families to split and divide, there are common themes that are worth noting.

The importance of parental self-esteem

I believe that the greatest asset anyone can have to defend against the onset of addiction is self-esteem. Most parents seek to endow their children with this valuable asset. But how can you teach it unless you have it yourself? How can you expect someone to respect you if you don't respect yourself? The relationship you have with yourself is reflected in your other relationships. Some people really do need to learn to love themselves a bit more, and many of those people I find are the parents of the children or teens who are presenting with an addictive disorder. This might be a coincidence but what I have found over the years is that when the parent develops a more loving relationship with themselves the impact on their relationship with their children improves commensurately.

Whenever I talk about 'loving yourself', people react with awkwardness and embarrassment, perhaps dismissing my suggestion as 'hippy speak' or 'happy-clappy nonsense', as if seeking to shame me into silence. Some imitate a version of loving yourself that might be more akin to narcissism – the original Narcissus staring into his reflection as Echo hovers nearby watching in adoration. This reaction to the word 'love' is worth exploring because a parent's personal experience of love is likely to affect the love that they give their child, and if that is awkward, ashamed, fearful or adoring then what impact is it having? It is certainly not the love, or self-love, that you might seek to promote.

Self-love

I am not suggesting you look at yourself in the mirror, 80s-style, and give yourself a wink of admiration. That kind of narcissistic self-love is not what I'm advocating here. Rather I am interested in a loving, honest and forgiving relationship with yourself so that you can accept your human-ness, learn from your mistakes and appreciate your and others' efforts. I believe that this kind of self-love can inspire, reflecting a compassionate relationship with yourself which will include care, nurture, understanding and forgiveness as well as boundaries and constructive criticism. If you care about yourself, you will treat yourself in a way that shows that you know you matter, and from this place you ask for respect in all that you do: around your space, your views and your interest. This is not do as I say but do as I do – you practise what you preach. From a position of self-love, in this way, you will find you are less threatened by others' views and behaviours, including those of your children and their friends, and that instead you are more tolerant and much less open to being manipulated.

If you know yourself and your history and recognise how these things play out in your parenting, then you are well on your way to being able to take responsibility for who you are as a parent.

Parental influence

Usually the pathway into my consulting room is littered with resentments and failed attempts at making changes, so it's often hard to come in and talk. Polarised views have been established, roles attributed around who is right and who is wrong, and very often there is what I would call an enmeshment, a relationship that is too close, intertwined so that it is hard to see one person as distinct from the other. In order to begin to sort out the family dynamics I need to first separate the various components, being each family member, assess and appreciate what each of those compo-nents is made of – family history, current circumstances – and then look at how they might all inter-react so that we have a better chance of success. In order to do this, I revert to frameworks that help me standardise my approach and one of those is to consider the influence of each parent on each child. The way I think about it is that the same gender parent is key to the development of identity and 'self' in the child, and the opposite gender parent is most influential in how that child translates into the world. Or simply put: same gender is how I feel about myself, and opposite gender is how I feel about you, the world and how I expect you experience me. I would also include older siblings in this framework as representative of the same pattern so that same gender affect identity, self-worth, etc. and opposite gender affect relationship with the world (whether I expect to be understood, liked, appreciated and what and who I am attracted to – or not!). Knowing how you impact your child is important.

. . . .

Gerard was very worried about his teenage son, Theo. He described Theo as academic, loyal, with huge potential and ambition, but presenting with repeated social difficulties so that he had moved schools twice as a result of bullying since year 8. Gerard described a close relationship with his son and seemed to feel overtly responsible for these difficulties. Willing to attend therapy on his own or with Theo, Gerard asked for an appointment. Meeting Theo and interviewing him privately, I discovered that he was indeed close to his father and seemed present with good self-esteem and a solid sense of his own potential. However, when he described his mother, Theo described a relationship fraught with difficulty as her volatile temper and self-destructive moods had often come his way in the form of threats, shaming accusations and violent outbursts, where plates were smashed and doors slammed. Theo was tearful, clearly feeling guilty as he felt he had betrayed his mother by talking about his experience in her care. But it didn't surprise me, as his difficulties manifested in his relationship with others, which in my view is reflected in the relationship with opposite gender parent. I spoke to Gerard, who confirmed his wife's mental health difficulties around anxiety and depression, but he felt she would be willing to attend therapy, which she did. It took a handful of sessions, first with the mother, Salli, so that she was able to work through and understand her behaviour without blame. Here she learned how to be accountable to Theo without interpreting his experience as her being a 'bad mother', but instead hearing him and how his experience of her had affected him. Salli's way of showing her apology then, after verbally doing so, was to be there for him in a way that she felt proud of and Theo was able

*to begin to rely on. There was a moment in session where Theo
was really quite blaming and I saw Salli look at me, hurt and
afraid for a moment of the power of his resentment. She took her
cue from me, reminded that all she was there to do was to listen,
which is what she did. At the next session, he apologised for how
he had spoken to her, but held onto his truth. She was held to
account, and it felt fair. They have never looked back.*

Just in case it sounds like I'm advocating being an emotional punchbag for
your child in order to pay penance for any mistake, I am not. The work
Salli did prior to going into session with Theo was to find peace with
herself about her own behaviour, which means she went into that session
with her son with understanding and self-respect. Thus, Salli could hear
him without becoming defensive and without becoming the hurt child or
teenager wanting attention and fearing rejection. Instead she could be there
as a mother for him, and for herself as the mother she wanted to be.

Sibling influence

Siblings are the original peer group that help socialise the child. Whatever
messages that are learned here will be taken forward into all the social
relationships, so that if a girl's older brother bullies her, for example, she is
likely to go on to seek out the same and then toughen up in an attempt to
become immune and not let any other male close to her. If a sibling is hurt
or ill in some away, the other siblings are likely to compensate by either
being super demanding or needless and wantless. When a parent is not
able, for whatever reason, to fulfil the parental role, often the oldest child
will take up position as 'parentifed child', so that the other siblings turn to
them as a kind of alternate parent. This can create overt expectation on that
older child that they are unable to meet because they are simply not old or
mature enough, and so they end up taking the brunt of the displaced disappointment and loss that was really the responsibility of the parent. This can
leave the parentifed child feeling deeply resentful and misunderstood.

In each family, there is a different puzzle and here I'd like to encourage your curiosity to become interested in the one that is yours. The process of socialising and establishing how you fit in the world can begin to happen within these sibling relationships, minefields riddled with power play, and hierarchies that include envy, competition and rejection, as much as connection and intimacy.

Envy

A powerful influence that is often overlooked because admitting being envious can leave you feeling insecure and/or less than, and to admit being the object of envy can sound boastful or invite criticism. An envious older sibling or parent can crush a child's confidence to be themselves for fear of upsetting the family member. Thus in response to sibling or parental envy, a person might dumb down, or self-sabotage, so fearful are they of being hated or ostracised just for being themselves.

As parents, it's easy to fall into the trap of attributing positive characteristics such as 'the clever one', 'the funny one', 'the sporty one' to each child, often with the intent of being fair. But in so doing you can paint your child into a corner where they can get stuck. From here it might be hard to try something new, especially if the new thing is the domain of another sibling. Better to allow the child to grow and develop as a person and keep the external experiences as interchangeable and common ground, available for sharing and connection, rather than as ways to cement identity.

The right motivation

It is a weekly event for me to witness yet another teenager roll their eyes as their parent leans forward to tell them that all they want is for them to be happy. Of course, there is nothing wrong with wanting your child to be happy, but this statement generally only serves to infuriate.

It's tough trying to motivate anyone to do something they're not sold on, but especially when it's a teen you're trying to convince. Part and parcel of being a teenager is to reject the advice of your parents, so it's a fine line you walk in advice-giving.

I don't often meet a teen whose motivation is to be happy so their parent can be pleased. Conversely, what I have seen time and again is a teen deny what he does want just to thwart parental expectation. Perhaps the right motivation then is a selfish one, which, if coupled with good self-esteem, is more likely to be a healthy and productive one.

Start by respecting your teen so that you actually listen to where they are coming from and how they see things. Listening doesn't give them power or make them right, it should simply make you closer. It might even change your point of view. Try not to exploit their vulnerability. If they open up to you, try not to dive in. Pace yourself and show faith and trust that this opening up can keep happening. Try to hear what your teenager actually wants. You may have ambitions for them, but this might cloud your view as to who they are or at least who they think they are or what they're capable of. The right motivation for the child is a selfish one so that they can own whatever they are doing. Your motivation is that it is healthy and productive.

How to manage stress – yours and others

When stress isn't managed, it's likely to be displaced onto other people. It happens all the time in road rage or in crowds, where people ventilate their built-up frustration through personal attack. In the home, children are an easy target as recipients of any of the emotions a parent or primary caregiver doesn't manage well. If the parent arrives home stressed out, the child may have to do very little to bear the brunt of that built-up stress. From approximately nought to six years old, the child is set up to soak up their environment without defence. After that, the frontal cortex of the brain becomes the dominant filter for all information so the child processes in a more conscious way. All these experiences shape the brain, which in turn shape the child's future relationships with others as well as with themselves.

So it's important to learn how to better handle your stress and realise how important it actually is not to dump it on somebody else. It can feel heavy and very unfair to receive.

Many of my clients are under tremendous pressure either because of the ambition of their work or because of the need simply to earn to keep the family together. On returning home, they are often hurrying back to take on the childcare, while work is not completely done for the day, so they are still on their phones, answering emails or finishing some sort of business as they walk through the door. But as I often tell these parents, the minute you walk through the door, you are Mum or Dad, your professional identity gone, your children will demand from you as a parent and you need to be ready, and even grateful for it. To be angry and frustrated at their seeming lack of respect or recognition that you have 'only just got in from work' or have 'had a tough day' or to wait until 'this important call is finished' is to betray your role as parent and to overlap the work boundary into the home, and this is your responsibility to manage, not theirs. My advice would be to switch off from work in whatever form that takes as you return home. Try:

1. Communicating to work that you will not be available for the first thirty minutes to one hour when you get home.
2. Put down your phone as soon as you get home for that first time period (don't keep it on your person, commit to being at home).
3. Make sure that you complete all urgent emails/calls before you turn into your street – give yourself at least fifteen minutes to breathe and let go and be just you before walking through your front door.
4. Tell your children how much time they have with you – be clear and maintain the boundary. Remember the importance of quality over quantity – if they have enough of you in a focused way they will more easily move onto something else.
5. Be grateful to be reminded of why you are working so hard and for the demands of your children as they greet you. It

might keep you grounded as you might be the CEO at work, but here you are Mummy or Daddy – be glad of it, there's only one of you!

How to manage your child's moods

The first step in managing your child's mood is to model a healthy relationship with your own mood. This should include the entire repertoire of emotion so that you experience all feelings in a healthy enough way, and when things go wrong, you own it and try and learn better for next time. This shows your child how to have the wide range of emotion available to us as humans in relationship with one another, and also how to make mistakes and move on. When I meet a teenager who tells me that they have never seen their mother or father angry or sad, then I expect that teenager to have difficulty around those very emotions. I have also seen teenagers present with extreme anger to a parent who admits that they are conflict averse, and I don't believe that this is a coincidence. It seems to me that a child will often demand the very thing from their parent that the parent struggles with as if demanding their parent deal with their most private weakness.

It is not helpful when a parent is afraid of their child's mood and an effort has to be made to reassert the appropriate hierarchy that puts parents back in charge in a respectful way. Managing your child's mood when you are afraid or feel out of your depth will give the message to your child that they are too much or perhaps that they are in charge, both dangerous messages that can cause trouble later. You feeling out of your depth is usually a reaction born of deeper influences than just your child's behaviour. I read somewhere that 'parents get children they deserve' and I have always found this to be an interesting if uncomfortable thought to reflect on in difficult times!

How to avoid behaving in ways that cause you to feel ashamed

In order to maintain self-respect, and to be able to demand respect by default from your child it is vital that you do not allow yourself to deteriorate into disrespectful behaviour that you later might feel ashamed of. Often when this happens the parent seeks to justify their behaviour by describing how badly the child behaved to trigger it, and their partner will be put in the difficult positon of having to choose who was the bad/good guy in the exchange. Was it the child who caused the parental behaviour or is the parent's behaviour the parent's responsibility?

The truth is we are all responsible for our own behaviour, especially when we are parents, and it will serve us all well to remember that we reap what we sow! There is a difference between feeling angry, for example, and acting out in our anger, and it is the latter that I think most parents need support around. Bringing up children is not easy; it requires you to be in good enough shape yourself to handle the various projections and displacements that inevitably come your way as a result of being a parent, and with all the various pressures we face today as single parents, working and with children who have more freedom than ever before, these pressures can feel relentless and time can feel short. So it is not without empathy that I, as a single parent with three children, acknowledge this challenge.

Actions:

When you feel annoyed with your child, try to:

- Notice how you feel before you act.
- Remember how old your child is and remind yourself of the power you have.
- Be the person you want to be – focus on how you feel about yourself and how you want to feel in, for example, thirty minutes, as much as your desire to control your child.
- Remember you're in this for the long haul – sometimes smaller, firm actions make more of a difference than a big gesture.
- Make the time to do whatever you need to do properly and kindly – taking the time now saves time later.

Technology – a great present for an argumentative future!

So many parents are at their wits' end, exasperated to the point of a kind of madness as a result of their interactions with their teenager and technology. The scenario plays out something like this: a parent calls to the teen to join them for supper and there is no answer. The parent then goes to find their child only to discover them engrossed in a PlayStation or Xbox game. A now more urgent repeat of the word 'supper' prompts irritation from the teenager, who is connected to their game with such single-minded attention it excludes all else, causing the parent to become annoyed, challenging the game and confronting what they consider to be their teen's rudeness prioritising 'that stupid game' over a basic need such as supper (which the parent has spent time preparing). At this point, the teen is likely to wave the parent away, dismissive and increasingly annoyed at the disruption of parental intrusion, which in turn causes the parent to ramp up their challenge. This exchange can increase in intensity and aggression in milliseconds, so that both teenager and parent end up shouting at each other, and it's not unusual for the parent (in their belief that they should be in control and their exasperation at a perceived lack of respect) to become physical with their teen, wrestling the controller out of their hand or engaging in push and shove to turn the machine off. I have even heard of gaming consoles or TVs being thrown out of windows! Now the teenager will turn to look at the adult with contempt (and probably a degree of fear), believing the entire problem to be the parent's behaviour, and the parent will feel forced to justify their behaviour, no matter how shocked or guilty they feel.

What is actually happening here?

Games are made to be addictive, we know this. It is deliberate on the part of the games designers to make them incredibly difficult to put down or pause. As parents we need to understand and respect this – our children and teens can experience an emotional and psychological charge in a similar way to someone using a class A stimulant drug when they are engaged in these games. Thus when you intervene, they overreact. Usually when I speak to the teen privately at another time, I discover that they do know they were meant to come off the game or to stop but they couldn't, and they often feel bad and uncomfortable about this, and then sometimes become interested about the impact the gaming is having on them. But in the instance described above, the parent has allowed themselves to pick up the tab so that instead of the child or teen feeling like they have done something wrong, or that they are agitated because of the game, in their view it's the parent that is the problem – because it was.

What needs to happen here?

The child or teenager needs to experience the consequences of their relationship with the gaming in terms of their agitation, aggression or intolerance without the parent getting caught up in the middle and that requires careful footwork. Some simple guides include pointing out what's going on and then not sticking around to be the target of the displacement. But that 'pointing out' needs to be delivered with care and sincerity not sarcasm and provocation; you're pointing it out because you care and you're in it for the long game. If you get angry or lose your temper, then you become the problem, not the gaming!

Questions:
Imagine in your mind's eye where you are positioned as you discipline or affirm your child.
- Are you metaphorically wagging your finger?
- Are you standing hands on hips?
- Do you have your arms out ready to catch your child as you believe they will they inevitably fall?
- Or have you got your back turned with your arms crossed?
- Where are you positioned in relation to the child you are experiencing so much difficulty with?

Stand shoulder to shoulder so you are close, supportive and advisory without being judgemental or overly involved (you have your own life, they have theirs). Try not to react, stay open and interested – fake it to make it and really try as you do not want to deepen a rift.

Comment simply and then step away – don't get drawn into answering their justifications.

If you do need to talk to your child try not to sit opposite across the table, but instead position yourselves one on the end and one on the side so that you are shoulder to shoulder as you discuss whatever the problem is.

Actions:

Just before you go to tell your child off or to address their behaviour, ask yourself how you feel.

- Think about what you want to teach not only in what you want to say, but in how you say it – do you want to shame your child or help them to take responsibility?
- Remember how you feel about yourself when you have made a mistake.
- Consider all that you have already read and learned about how much influence you have in how you deliver a message.
- What will help you get to a respectful shoulder-to-shoulder position – perhaps it might be to recall some of your own mistakes?
- Remember the good things in your child to counterbalance the fury you might feel at them right now.
- Remember that affirming a child and showing them patience as they learn teaches them to do the same.
- Keep your message simple and focus on the behaviour; don't make it personal.
- You can feel angry without being angry . . .

10

BOUNDARIES AND RULES

You *have* boundaries, you put up walls

A boundary, in my view, is a representation of an individual's personal relationship with themselves and the world that relates to their moral code, social expectation, social interaction and communication. If a person has boundaries they have self-respect. This is not about controlling another, it's about representing self in such a way it might inspire behaviour in another. These boundaries relate to aspects of a person that include their emotions, sex, thoughts and behaviours, and can be internal or external, the purpose of which is to protect and represent self (and sometimes other) as well as to connect.

Boundaries allow somebody to feel safe because the person with the boundaries knows where they stand with themselves, and what they will or won't accept from someone else; they also know how they will react to any violation of the boundary. There is a confidence in somebody who has good boundaries that is comfortable to be around. It's as if they know where they start and end; therefore, it is easier to figure out where you are in relation to them. Also when a person protects themselves with boundaries, they prevent themselves from becoming a victim, which is an act of self-esteem, allowing intimacy in good mutual knowledge while taking personal responsibility.

A lack of boundaries is present where there is inconsistency so that rules and expectations can change according to mood, personality or circumstance. Also where relationships are too close and identities and roles blurred, for instance when people are enmeshed or in relationships driven by fear of intimacy and avoidance. The apparent clarity of the all-or-nothing reaction indicates a lack of moderation and no boundaries.

Rules are explicit messages and guidelines that require observation usually in order to maintain social structure, safety and effective, respectful communication. Rules that are not observed will have consequences that should be followed through. Rules are an externalised message that may have evolved from a boundary. Rules simply allow somebody to know what's expected of them, usually in terms of behaviour, and what the consequences will be if they are not followed. Thus, there is safety in knowing where you stand in relation to constructive rules that you can then choose to follow or not, either by taking an educated risk, by sheer defiance, through conforming or maybe you agree with the rule because it just makes sense. Transparent, reasonable rules are a cornerstone of any civilised society whether that's on a macro scale or in a micro sense within a family.

Certainly with teenagers, you can expect your rules to be broken, brink-manship to be part of the relationship and consequences will need to be followed through. However, boundaries should not be exploited or violated as this will cause personal offence and hurt that can often be difficult to repair. It is important to understand the difference between the two.

Examples of boundaries

- to treat one another with respect
- to listen to one another (without pulling faces, even a little bit, and without prepping your answer!)
- to be honest with one another
- to learn how to compromise so that any solution is less often black/ white, win/lose but more collaborative, taking into account one another's needs
- use words to represent yourself, and to give one another the time to gather their thoughts and express themselves
- not to shout, threaten, dominate

- to apologise when necessary, and to consider that apology without shaming or seeking power
- to ask for time if you need it; to give time if it's asked for
- to be curious rather than take things personally so that you are offended
- to be curious about your own responses instead of reacting without reflection
- to respect your own and the other person's emotional/intellectual process
- not to physically hurt yourself or anyone else, even as a result of how you feel
- to say no when you need to; to protect yourself from e.g. becoming overwhelmed or overstretched (and therefore resentful)
- to acknowledge your own humanity and forgive yourself your mistakes and commit to learning from them
- to consider your needs and wants and take care of those as a priority so that you are in a position to give without conditions
- to allow yourself to experience pleasure as a natural, human need
- to allow yourself to refuse unhappy or damaging experiences

Examples of rules for teenagers

- don't drink and drive
- don't get in the car if the driver is drunk
- lock the door when you come in
- return home by (X) o'clock
- get out of bed by (X) o'clock
- make your bed every day
- put your dishes in the dishwasher
- put your washing out
- tidy your room
- no phones at mealtimes
- no smoking in the house

Boundary violations include

- Yelling or screaming, ridiculing and shaming, attempting to control or manipulate, interrupting, blaming
- Physically they include getting too close or touching without permission, and this includes sexual contact, touching another person's belongings, reading a diary without permission or listening into a private conversation
- Smoking around non-smokers and exposing someone else to something contagious
- Demanding unsafe sexual practices or insisting and engaging in a particular sexual act irrespective of the other person's resistance

Difficulty delivering a rule or consequence?

When delivering a message to your child or teenager, it is important to remember that there are two key components to consider that will influence the effectiveness of the delivery. The first is how the child or teenager feels about the message itself and the second is how the child or teenager feels about you.

On the first point, I often refer to children as 'heat-seeking missiles for what they want' and you are in the way of what they want or the means to getting what they want. On the second point, too often a child can shoot the messenger and distort how the message is heard or even plays out, and this is usually because they don't respect that parent, perhaps only on that point or sometimes sadly across the board.

Most children will do all they can to get life on their terms and to get their own way. This is natural. They will push, threaten, cajole and manipulate. If the parent gives in at any point they are confirming the child is in charge. This makes it ever harder to say 'no' to this child the next time, causing the child to persist in seeking the usual 'magic button' when they get their way. The more this happens, the more determined they will get. If as a parent you cannot handle anger then that is the button the child will push when you refuse; if it's tears you can't deny, then it's tears you will get. The key is that once you have said 'no', and it's important you have thought about it before you do so and the 'no' comes from a respectful considered place, then you are no longer talking about the thing you said 'no' about, you are teaching acceptance and confronting self-will. Holding this boundary of a 'no' can precipitate an apology from the child for their outburst and at this point many parents capitulate, believing it's important to affirm their child's self-awareness – but it is more likely to be an awareness of what the parent needs to see for the child to get their way! At this stage, maintain the boundary and affirm the acknowledgement and resourcefulness the child is showing even if it is to get their own way – but hold the boundary, and be prepared to go through it all again. Acceptance of life on life's terms is a quality I rarely see, on intake anyway, so the exercise on page 176 is well worth practising.

Splitting

An increasingly misused term, 'splitting' actually describes the inability to hold both negative and positive aspects of an entity or person in one place so that instead the perception becomes 'good' and 'bad', as in the case of parents, where there is one perceived as each rather than both being both and human. Often developing as a result of early trauma, the child compartmentalises in order to cope and feel secure, thinking in absolute terms rather than the less definitive grey area. If your child is prone to this kind of splitting, it may be worthwhile seeking a therapist to help them to cope with their polarised views of the world which will otherwise potentially set them up for conflict and maybe even a need within themselves to self-medicate. As the experience of trauma is likely to be early, I would suggest EMDR as a possible approach because it has a direct effect on the way the brain processes information and allows you to move through the 'frozen' feeling people get when they are stuck in cyclical behaviours. I think the difference even in the language of describing an experience as 'splitting' or 'divide and rule' is important to notice, as the latter suggests a sense of intent and agency, whereas the other sounds divisive and might leave a parent feeling manoeuvered.

Usually when parents talk about 'splitting' they are talking about the 'divide-and-rule' strategy that many children will use to get what they want. They will employ this tactic again and again, especially if it works. Remember, children are heat-seeking missiles for what they want and you are often the only thing that's in the way, so brace yourself!

It is inevitable that parents will have differing views on many subjects and it is how this difference is managed that is important: there's nothing wrong with a child knowing that there's more than one approach or one view or one answer. The problem lies when the child is able to exploit the difference between the two views because the result of that will be a lack of respect and what might be called a falsely empowered child. This is relatively easy to handle when the child is under eleven, but the teen years will be when you pay the debt.

Whether you are together or separate, as parents it is useful when your child asks you for something to check if they have already asked the other parent and, if they have, to ask what the response was. Of course, this doesn't apply to absolutely everything but it is a useful technique to instill as second nature because it shows recognition and respect between the parents.

Where there is a persistent difference of opinion between parents, if you can't sort it out between yourselves, each of you simply has to accept that you must agree to disagree. In this climate, your child will also learn that both parents believe themselves to be right, and so they learn there is no such thing as one answer. The frustration here is often that one parent feels forced into a more disciplinary role because the other has adopted a lenient or indulgent position. What's useful to remember here is that as a parent you should not compensate for the other parent's behaviour. Figure out what your view is, explore why you cannot agree with the other parent and why some sort of compromise isn't possible, and then in your own right represent your view with dignity and respect. If your child is at an age where they can understand and make decisions for themselves, then they are likely to choose the one that suits them best. This might anger you if you are trying to do the best thing for your child and you are confounded by an indulgent other half or ex, but sometimes there is nothing you can do. If you let your anger get the better of you, it not only represents you in an angry light, but you are likely to further alienate your child. This may seem grossly unfair, but relief comes in the literature from the anonymous fellowships whereby step one is an acceptance of powerlessness of other people, places and things. All we can do is our best. Don't give up your dignity for anyone or anything.

Teaching acceptance

When I think about the one thing that is rarely present in anyone seeking help at my practice, it is the acceptance of life on life's terms, as most people I meet are living on their terms, even if it's hurting them. The exercise on page 176 about being able to say 'no' is important in teaching acceptance.

The concept of powerlessness as touched on above too is so alien to most people that I meet because they have engaged, sometimes for years, in patterns of seeking solutions, short-term fixes and attempts to control that have backfired so that relationships, physical health, finances and prospects have suffered, sometimes beyond repair. Thus it seems to me that teaching your child a sense of acceptance that challenges entitlement, fosters integration but is delivered with respect is key to the entire prevention message. I'm hoping it is also accessible for you to replicate from this brief description.

As discussed throughout this book, the first and most important position is to ensure that the parent or primary caregiver is in good shape. I cannot reiterate this point enough as the quality of the source of any information or interaction has a massive effect on how it is received and applied. As parents you matter a very great deal and, in my view, to survive the teen years and come out the other side still close is a big challenge. Practising self-care as an integral part of your daily discipline will help with this as it requires you to care about yourself enough to take care of your needs. If you do this in small, integrated ways you will not only model the same behaviour to your children, but you will also make your life so much easier.

Be good enough

Having respect for boundaries, yours and those of your family, will help you feel like a 'good enough parent'. It will mean that you listen without being defensive because you're interested in the other person's point of view. It means when you speak you're not pointing fingers, just expressing yourself so that you may be known. If you manage to stand in your own esteem you will model dignity and respect regardless of whether what you say and do meet with your child's approval.

When bringing up children, it's useful to have three answers at your fingertips to respond to the infinite and relentless demands of your offspring. These need to be 'yes', 'no' and 'I don't know'. 'Yes' is unlikely to cause you any emotional or relational difficulties with your child, 'no' can be like stepping on a mine and 'I don't know' is only effective if your child knows you have a robust 'no' in your repertoire. If they don't, then your 'I don't know' will prompt endless badgering and insistent negotiations as they believe you will inevitably give in and say 'yes'. Learning how to say 'no' and holding that boundary will deliver you the relief that an 'I don't know' can provide. This is definitely worth learning.

If you're feeling under pressure from your child, it's probably because you haven't expressed or shown clearly enough your personal boundary, so this needs to be done. For example, a falsely empowered child who pushes their parents around and gets their own way will often feel strangely insecure, believing nothing can contain them, distrusting authority figures and maybe bullying or finding someone who is a bully who can contain (control) them, thereby providing the safety (which is far from safe) they crave. At the other end of the scale, the child may feel ashamed if they are told all their demands are upsetting the parent. These children are at risk of shutting down and becoming dangerously in denial of their own needs, instead developing an internalised rage.

It's so important that the parent can contain the child, respectfully. So even if it makes you feel angry, you don't have to *be* angry when you assert that boundary or stand by it when it's tested. Just follow the message through.

Questions:

- Can you say 'yes' or 'no' to your child?
- If not, what are you afraid is going to happen?
- Do you know why you think this will happen?
- How can you consciously challenge this thinking, so all three answers are available to you as a parent ('yes'/'no'/'I don't know')?

When you say 'no' to a child or a teenager, they will be dropped into an experience of loss. This is because much of the time when they ask for something, in their head they've already got it. Whether that's a new iPhone, a party they want to go to, shopping trip or sleepover, believe you me, before they've asked you for permission they've researched on the Internet which model they want, already discussed it with their friends, planned what they're going to wear, know what they want to buy . . . the only thing that's in the way is you! So no matter how innocuous the approach, the minute you say 'no', the battle is on.

It's useful to be aware of the grief and loss stages conceptualised by Elisabeth Kübler-Ross (1969): denial, anger, bargaining, depression, acceptance. In this model I have adapted them so that they are as follows:

Stages of grief and loss

- **Shock:** This is the sharp intake of breath, the disbelief sometimes articulated by arm gestures or a retort such as 'what?' or 'I don't get why you're saying that . . .'
- **Denial:** In line with this model, denial takes the form of argument, denying the fact and converting it into something else so that there is some purchase on the point, e.g. universalising (everybody does it / has one / is going), minimising (it's not such a big deal), exaggerating (why do you always have to be so negative) etc.
- **Anger:** The outburst, outrage, shouting, swearing, accusing, walking out and slamming a door, e.g. 'I hate this house and I

hate you', 'you never listen to me, you just don't care' or 'you're ruining my life'.

- **Sadness:** The tears that come sometimes as a result of the relief following anger, sometimes in place of anger, and sometimes from genuine sadness. There is a breakdown into hopelessness and self-pity.
- **Negotiation/bargaining:** Having walked out, the child may return to the scene of the argument with an apology for how they have spoken and behaved, recognition of the impact this has on the parent, and a negotiation that if they do their homework on Friday not Sunday / walk the dog / contribute some money, etc. might the parent reconsider their answer.
- **Acceptance (or not):** This is where most people go wrong because they believe that the negotiating/bargaining stage shows that their child understands what they have done wrong and has learned a lesson. This is highly unlikely as all they have probably understood is what you want to hear from them so that they get their way. So the answer remains 'no' though you accept the apology. If they're trying to play you, you will go back through this process again and again in the hope that you will get worn down or lose it and then have to compensate. If they have learned from this process, then you will know . . . because it will die down.

Once you have said 'no', then you are teaching your child the 'life on life's terms' experience that there is such a thing as 'no', for good reason. The second part of the sentence is really important as it is not just 'no means no', but that you have listened to your child's request, considered it and come up with a respectful answer based on a rationale which they may or may not agree with, but which does exist. It's all very well to bring a child up to be resourceful and to be able to think around problems and not just give up, but that must be within the safety of a reasonable and consistent boundary that represents a recognition that we share this world with one another.

'I don't know' is a moment of pause when you're asked something by your child and it's not good timing nor do you have an immediate answer. But as I have already said this is only an option if your child knows that you have a 'no' that you are able to hold. Once that it is in place then 'I don't know, leave it with me' becomes a valid option. However, it is very important that you give a timeframe to a child within which you will return to them with an answer so they learn how to wait, respectfully.

As you seek to apply these techniques at home where it might already feel quite out of control, it might not immediately 'work' in the way you hope. In fact, things might get a lot worse before they get better. It makes sense though that if your child is used to getting what they want, even if that's a big row or something negative, then when you apply the technique that interrupts this process they will ramp up the pressure. In part this is in disbelief that you are changing and it's trustworthy, and secondly because they are used to getting their own way. As the pressure mounts it is important that you recognise the part you have played in creating the 'mini monster' in front of you so that, in recognition that you are part of this dynamic, you have some responsibility. Hopefully this delivers you with some patience.

You may find you go round and round the same grief and loss process and it's important that you learn just to stand still in the knowledge that you are no longer talking about the iPhone/party/shopping trip/sleepover . . . you are now trying to teach acceptance. I don't suggest you explain that, nor do I suggest that you do much else other than calmly reinforce your point. It should only be a matter of weeks before things start to improve.

What is also interesting to note is that each child will respond to each parent differently. When parents say that they brought their children up all the same and try to analyse each child as if the environment were a consistent one, they are at risk of overlooking a vital component that could deliver them with the insight that might help. Every child is different. Each parent is different. Each parent is different with every child and vice versa. Each child is born into a different dynamic and how you treat your first child is different to how you treat your second and so on. The first child is born without a sibling group. The second child creates a sibling group. The circumstances for the family change as life progresses in terms of geography, money, health, time, availability and also in terms of the relationship between mother and father. So many differences that are so often not taken into account as parents reflect.

Looking at the model above, I would advise each parent to note how each child reacts to each of them when a 'no' (or an 'I don't know') is delivered. Given that the child is determined to get what they want, they will not bother with the responses that don't work, especially with a parent who they have got to know intimately for the whole of their lives. Instead they will go straight for the response that delivers the result. Thus . . .

- if your child comes to you with shock as a first response, threatening in that sharp intake of breath the conflict that is to come, then it might be worth you exploring your fear of conflict that makes that the most effective response for them
- if the negotiation skills of denial kick in, then maybe you are someone who likes to argue the detail
- if your child responds with anger it is likely they have experienced anger from you themselves, so they match it or provoke it as it bears results, perhaps through the shame that often follows an angry outburst
- if they cry, then simply you would do well to explore why you struggle to cope with another's sadness – tolerating your child's pain is an important dimension of effective parenting

Questions:
You need boundaries to teach boundaries. Born of self-respect, boundaries speak for themselves. Delivering a rule with boundaries is likely to have a more successful outcome than without!
- How do I feel about my own time, space and needs?
- Do I make enough time for these in my life?
- Do I resent everyone else for leaving me running on empty?
- Do I feel I have the right to control how much people take from me emotionally or how close another person gets to me, including touching me or my personal property?
- How do I represent this?
- Do I extend the same respect to my child?

- Do I make demands of my child without respect?
- Does my child have good boundaries?
- Can he/she say no and mean it?
- Do I affirm him or her for their boundaries or do I resent them when they don't suit me?
- Can I say yes/no and I don't know and mean it?

As a working, single parent I know all too well the pitfalls and pain of timetabling family life alongside a demanding job. Often tired and under pressure, I might be easy prey for my children and their demands. The guilt of being a working mum is a place I can go to if I choose. But generally I don't. I know why I do what I do and I take responsibility for that.

It's important not to shirk from the truth because as parents, as you have already read, we do have a significant influence on a child's development through our own behaviours. It's worth remembering too that as you might seek to manipulate your child to do what you want, in a few years those very tricks may well come back to bite you!

Instead use boundaries, consistent clear boundaries, not to control the other person, but more as an influence, a guide, a kind of GPS signal that is consistent and trustworthy, emitted from you to the world. I like to think of it as a lighthouse, sending out a signal that is constant and true. These boundaries signify the demarcation of who you are, what is acceptable to you and what is not, what makes you laugh and what makes you sad, what interests you, what is appropriate and what is intolerable. It allows you to be truly known.

When a boundary is compromised it corrupts that signal, breaking your own moral code, and you will end up possibly lying or denying your own needs, manipulating, enabling and acting in ways that are not 'you'. The signal is 'lost' and those around you will feel it.

Questions:

- In what way do my boundaries reflect who I am?
- If I were to choose an image to help me maintain my boundaries, what would that be? For example, it could be a lighthouse. Find a picture that works for you and put it somewhere to remind you in times of difficulty.

11

HOW TO GET WELL AND STAY WELL

Be proactive: be the parent you want to be

Early intervention

If you think there is something wrong with your child, trust your gut and ask the question. If your child or teenager shuts you down, then I suggest you seek help from a relevant professional so that you can work out what is yours to process: your expectations, your unconscious fears and any unresolved patterns that might prejudice your ability to clearly assess your own children. Once you've done this you can re-enter your relationship in the family with your children and feel much more confident as you are clear where you start and end and they begin, which will allow you to challenge, support and intervene with less drama and confusion. Early intervention works. Getting somebody into therapy when they display the early signs of shame-based behaviour, low self-esteem or resentment is far better than waiting until they develop more sophisticated coping mechanisms that can set up a pattern of self-loathing in their own right, and can also be dangerous.

Damage

Of course as parents we do damage, how can we not when we are merely human and, for a while, so central to our children's world? We also do good, so remember that as you beat yourself up with your regrets. If you are solely responsible for the negatives your child displays then you must also be responsible for all the positives, too – of course, when you think about it rationally though, it isn't possible. I think taking the opportunity of addressing these patterns in yourself is to become less afraid of facing up to the damage we may have caused to our children as a result of our clumsy interventions. In facing up to them ourselves for being human (which lets our children off the expectation of being perfect themselves), and engaging in the living amend of change.

Each parent know yourself

As you will already have noticed, central to this philosophy is for each parent to do the work themselves before they impose it on another. Knowing and accepting yourself in glorious detail will allow you to understand why you react the way you do to certain triggers and more specifically, why you behave in certain ways when your children 'push your buttons'. Some people would cite table manners as of fundamental importance, and almost all those people I have ever spoken to with this etiquette as a value have had it drilled into them when they were young, or they suffered humiliation of some kind in relation to it. Everything comes from somewhere and knowing what your attentional bias is and why that might be allows you to choose to apply the same or a version of the same (or not) in your role as mother or father.

Avoid 'carried emotion'

Remember whenever we experience emotion as parents that we do not properly contain, our children by default are most likely to pick it up and convert it into 'carried emotion'. This can manifest negatively most commonly in terms of anxiousness, anger and shame, and they are hard to shift because quite often the child believes them to be their own. Thus an overanxious parent, not able to contain or reality check their own emotional experience, may become micro-managing, impatient or over-check every-thing, causing the child to shut down as they are unable to cope with the anxious attention. But within the withdrawal an anxiousness may take hold of the child, so that they too distrust and need to double-check or control, sometimes in apparently unrelated ways, such as by restricting food. Perhaps that parent is married to someone who is often angry – irritated by their partner's anxiousness, they are intolerant of the checking and make shameful statements about behaviour. The child watching this will begin to feel ashamed of their own self-doubt and fear the criticism, often converting this into anger onto themselves. When later they emerge as a perfectionist, with such low self-esteem that they never want to try for fear of failure, full of self-doubt and aggressive when approached with what the parent feels is constructive criticism, the parent should not be surprised. As I have said before – we reap what we sow – and it takes great courage to look at the ingredients we have put into our children's childhoods so that we can better understand and respectfully intervene.

An exercise in curiosity

Curiosity is an engaging quality that opens the window to the soul, allowing connection without offence. Being interested in what makes you tick can start a journey that builds self-esteem and a life you actually want to live. Notice what makes you laugh or cry, and then extend that to every emotion and into your boundaries without judging what is right or wrong, just so that you know yourself. What makes you annoyed or are your 'shoulds'? And be curious about your desire for justice, for example. Is it connected to an injustice from your childhood? Notice what you like to do or see or taste or touch. Wonder at who you like and what you are attracted to. Are these really your own tastes or have they been picked up from someone else? Are you allowed to be happy, or happy with yourself? How easily can you describe your self-image? (Maybe do a collage called 'me'.) Have a look at a picture of yourself aged five or six or seven and see if you can feel affection, because that child truly needs you to. Are you the kind of parent you wanted to be? And if you're not, what's got in the way? Does it have to stay that way?

I believe most of us want to be the best parent for our children's sake, but I would add that it is just as important for you to believe you're the best parent you can be for your own sake.

What is recovery from addiction?

Recovery is very different to sobriety as it is no longer about counting the sober days and more about making each day count. Recovery is a way of life that is respectful, curious, open and loving. As they say in the fellowship rooms – if you are **H**onest, **O**pen and **W**illing you are in the wrong place. HOW we get into recovery is to become all those things, but it will take time and that's OK. The marathon of early recovery is about eighteen months and then things start to consolidate, so take it step by step.

So many people resist accepting they are an addict for fear of the life sentence and negative stigma that label represents. But counter-intuitive though it may be, accepting that responsibility is exactly what sets you free as it lets you get hold of the solution with both hands.

Healthy selfish

The word selfish has so many negative connotations as it infers a neglect of another's needs or pattern of putting yourself first as if you were more important. But it is equally damaging to do the complete opposite and ignore your own needs in favour of everybody else's as you have already read. The middle ground is what you are looking for: this allows you to be as important as everybody else, neither better nor worse, and is where your needs must be evaluated by you so that you do not ever run on empty. Modelling this behaviour is the first vital influence in teaching it and the subsequent years reinforcing self-care as an important part of daily routine will help self-esteem. Healthy selfish means that when you are asked how you are, you think about it and give an appropriately truthful response. It doesn't mean saying 'I'm fine' when you're not, nor does it mean you pour your heart out to whomever asks. It means you represent yourself honestly with dignity and respect. Healthy selfish means that no matter another person's need you also need to achieve the basics of your self-care on a daily basis. Think carefully before you change your plans to accommodate somebody else's, especially if that person is somebody who quite often comes to you in a state of crisis. Are you sure setting your own needs to one side isn't enabling them to be unmanageable? Healthy selfish means you will be able to afford to be generous.

Rescue confirms victim

Giving somebody answers may feel like being helpful but what you are also doing is letting them know that you can see they can't do this on their own. In some circumstances, you might be right and your actions might actually be helpful but just as many times, giving someone answers can actually cause damage to self-esteem because the covert message is 'I can see you won't do this properly / understand this well enough / you're incapable'.

As a parent, it's hard to stand by and watch your children fight or argue but every time you step in you choose who is the victim and who is the persecutor, and your children see that as you taking sides. Sometimes it is better simply to let them know the impact that their arguing is having on you. Sometimes it's better to let them work it through. Instead of protecting the one who you feel is being attacked, tell the one attacking that you feel disappointed in them for behaving in that way and encourage them to find another way of expressing themselves. Change your focus and be proactive in your approach, extending your response to include all your children rather than playing referee. Don't tolerate it when it becomes physical – that is the time you need to intervene – but try to remain calm so that your children can experience the consequences of their behaviour instead of your feelings trumping everything.

Parent the good child too

It's completely natural for the attention to be drawn by the child who demands it by being sick, disruptive or angry. It's hard to remember to parent the child who is quiet or presents with few needs, and so many parents talk about being exhausted so they have nothing left for the other children let alone for each other. It's up to you as parents which child you respond to and how much time you give them. It's important to decide in advance for example how much time you're going to spend when you put each child to bed so that their presenting a drama to you as you tuck them up in bed doesn't ambush you. Instead you mark the issue and commit to talking about it another time. Make that time specific and follow through on making it happen.

It's important to affirm good behaviour, to acknowledge the gaps as well as the action, meaning noticing and commenting when somebody is quiet. When a child finds that being disruptive gets some attention even if it's negative attention, they will often continue to do it so that the parent is completely controlled by the child. This whole model is about the parent reclaiming the driving seat and having the space and time to decide whatever their response needs to be instead of just reacting in the moment to whatever stimulus.

The place of creativity

Children are very creative and it is part of a healthy developmental process to explore their world and use their imaginations. Encouraging this through playing games, arts and crafts and even telling stories can richly expand a child's capacity for thinking and understanding. The old saying that families who play together stay together is very true because in play, relationships are formed, and the family dynamic is understood and appreciated through the lens of having fun instead of always through the practicality of running a family home. It's really worth making sure that every week you do something with your child or your children that taps into this experience of play and creativity as it will reward you in the future tenfold.

Top and bottom lines

In rehab, bottom lines are how we describe the things people decide not to do anymore, like not going to pubs or other places where there is alcohol, not walking down a street that an ex-boyfriend lives on, or a dealer; some 'bottom line' eye contact with strangers, or eating sugar, or eating after 8 p.m.; some 'bottom line' contact with a friend or a family member. Bottom lines in early recovery can seem extreme, but they are there as visible guides to maintain safety until someone can learn to do this instinctively for themselves.

Written out in specific detail, there is no grey area to negotiate to try and get away with a slip or relapse. With drugs and alcohol for an addict, a bottom line is abstinence. For someone with an eating disorder, a bottom line would be to stick to their food plan. But too often we forget to bank the good stuff so it's important to have goals as well and remember what you want from all of this. This is called 'topline behaviours'. Remember to put in time for the things you enjoy, like spending time together or doing things that are fun – and make sure they happen.

Some ideas for topline behaviours

Watch a movie together, talk about feelings and what's going on together, sing or dance together, tell each other jokes, hug, leave each other notes when you go out, don't forget to thank each other, go for a walk or bike ride, lie in the grass and make shapes and stories out of the clouds, play a game of ball or tag or go to try a new sport together, do some volunteering, spend time outside and play in the park or in a woodland, go camping, have a go at their PlayStation or Xbox games with them, read the same books and talk about them, play memory games, cook, de-clutter or redecorate a bedroom or play space and never forget to say 'I love you'. It's worth knowing that spending non-competitive time together as parent and child, just getting to know one another, is priceless and will stand your relationship in good stead.

Enabling

Every addict will have an enabler (or two) nearby, who acts as an emotional dustpan and brush, a shock absorber soaking up their painful consequences, alleviating the pain. The advice to any enabler is that you should step out of the way as soon as possible so that the addict can experience the consequences of their behaviour, so that those consequences can teach them. If you cushion the blow, they will never learn because they don't have to. If you pay their debt for them, you enable the next expense. If you explain their mistakes away, they never have to face them. Enabling your child to abdicate responsibility by answering for them is a dangerous path to follow. It may feel like love, but you might be killing your child with kindness and indulging them or teaching them learned helplessness instead. Believing in someone is an affirmation and it manifests as a behaviour whereby you stand by their side – actually or metaphorically – and trust and support them by bearing witness as they experience their life.

Enmeshment

This can have a similar feel to enabling as there is a degree of rescue involved. But more specifically enmeshing with someone means you intertwine your life and thoughts and feelings with them so the line that separates you both is unclear. Often driven by an insecure parent who needs to be needed, the child is made to feel very special, which initially feels wonderful, but evolves to feeling suffocating and inhibiting.

Where this happens between parent and child, it makes separation and the maturing process extremely difficult so that if the child were to grow up and become independent they would have to reject the parent, which often they feel they cannot do. Instead the child might develop a pattern of addiction to warp the maturation process, and to justify the parent's closeness by needing them, while at the same time keeping them at a distance. The very nature of the addiction isolates the child from feeling too close.

The work here is to create the space for each person to establish their own identify and reset the boundary between them at a healthy distance. For example, if people were represented by circles in a Venn diagram, they should only overlap so that the greater proportion remains individual. In enmeshed relationships, one circle can completely obscure the other, so that one person gives up their identity to please the other.

Letting go

This doesn't mean turning your back on someone: it means realising and accepting your own powerlessness, and this should feel like a relief! There are some things you cannot do for someone else and there is some pain you cannot carry in place of another. Letting go allows others to have their own experiences instead of your version of their experiences. Letting go means you can be there and support someone as they grow and learn, without the judgement that notes what needs to be fixed and instead with empathy. Letting go enables them to do the work on themselves not you, so that their successes are their own, as are their failures. Letting go is about acceptance and allowing each day to come with curiosity and an open mind. Letting go is an act of love.

How to promote well-being so it is second nature

Practise, practise, practise . . . make patterns of self-care and well-being part of everyday life so that you show it, you all live it and your children learn it by osmosis until they can maintain it for themselves. It needs not to be a chore or a point of conflict, it just is. At first it might all seem too much, but once you get used to it, it will become part of everyday living

Mental well-being

Try to encourage your child to become interested in their own and others' thoughts and points of view by asking them what they think and by listening and reflecting. You don't have to agree, but you do have to be interested. You want to teach them to be curious and that happens when trying or saying something doesn't leave them feeling ridiculed or wrong. Open questions work well so the answer isn't a yes/no, but fuller. Say 'yes' when they want to talk to you, even if you're busy. Encourage conversation about things they have read or seen or experienced and see if they have a point of view and why. It will help you to know them and them to know themselves.

Physical well-being

There is no point in taking care of the mind if you don't learn to take equal care of the body.

1. **Food:** Make sure you and your child eat regularly and healthily as a cornerstone of physical well-being, such as three meals a day, including protein, fruit, veg and carbs, with portion sizes that roughly match the size of their fist. Notice what they eat and how they eat. Are they always in a hurry or is eating a time to enjoy and connect with others. Notice patterns of feeling hungry in case they are converting feelings into something physical, which can be a route to an eating disorder. It might feel much easier to feel hungry than face the fear of doing the essay, or of feeling fat instead of angry if anger isn't accepted in the household. In this day of technology, it's easy for children to let the hours slip by and only eat crisps or sweets – if this is happening, stop buying them until healthier snacks and eating routines have been put back in place and make sure the breaks happen.

2. **Exercise:** Mindful walking, swimming, being active, taking the stairs not the lift, joining an exercise, yoga or dance class, cycling – these are all healthy activities to incorporate into your child's life. Make sure that exercise isn't introduced as a way to control weight or mood, but as fun, and a healthy dimension to a productive life and for your child to 'stay in their shoes'.

3. **Self-care:** Washing, brushing teeth, tidying the bedroom, wearing clean clothes – all help reinforce healthy pride and self-esteem.

4. **Socialising:** We are social beings – make sure your child says 'yes' to a social event and develops relationships with friends. Socialising by virtual media is not enough! It's important too that you get to know parents as it helps cement the relationships between children.

5. **Stimulation:** Make sure your child does something that interests them or stimulates them physically, mentally and emotionally. Whether that's doing puzzles or reading a book, seeing a challenging movie or taking part in a physical activity. Keep them on their toes and keep them learning.

6. **Sleep:** Rest and sleep are two different things and sleep is essential for well-being as it's when our body recharges and cells regenerate so it literally keeps you well. Both you and your child need it! Government guidelines suggest:

   o Teenagers fourteen to seventeen years should have eight to ten hours of sleep

   o Young adults eighteen to twenty-five years should have seven to nine hours of sleep

   o Adults twenty-six to sixty-four years should have seven to nine hours of sleep

   o Older adults sixty-five years or older years should have seven to eight hours of sleep

   In order to sleep well we must practise sleep hygiene, which includes proper relaxation before falling asleep – the use of gaming technology and social media is counterproductive to that for one hour before lights out. Rest and relaxation are important de-stressing techniques that allow the body and mind to slow down, e.g. by having a hot bath, a nice meal, a good chat, watching a good movie. It is so hard to advise today's teenagers of all this, as they live with their phones attached to their heads, and gaming devices at their fingertips, but nonetheless it's true. So instead of saying 'I told you so' as they emerge exhausted from bed, try to support them into better self-care by expressing concern and then letting go. If you do the caring for them they will rebel. Your job is to help them to want to take better care of themselves as they are valuable. This will never happen if they have to agree that you're right!

7. **Feeling safe:** A child deserves to feel safe and to know this is their right. Teach this, promote this and honour this. Never compromise your child's safety by exposing them to someone or something dangerous. Drive safely and avoid road rage or displacing your feelings through your driving and drink driving. Teach them what is right so that they know and so that they can keep themselves safe.

Emotional well-being

Respect the fact that emotions exist and are immensely powerful as has been discussed throughout this book. Teaching a child how to have feelings safely and in a contained way takes time and patience, but it's a good investment. It's certainly easier too if you have a good relationship with your own emotional process first. At the back of this book there is a list of emotions for sadness, anger and shame – these are often the feelings that cause the most trouble. Find a way to help your child learn to have these feelings in a way that is safe and helpful.

1. Either as a parent or as a tool for your child, journalling is useful when you're going through difficult times so that you can express and then process the reality of what's going on instead of being trapped and convinced by your feelings.

. . . .

Joanna was prone to seeing things very negatively so she spent a month of simply marking each day as good, bad or indifferent (illustrated by emojis) at the beginning and end of every day. To her astonishment, even though she reported feeling low and hopeless

about her life in the therapy session, when she added up the marks
she had had a good month. Feelings are not facts.

The journal should note:
- What has happened.
- How you feel.
- What was going on before.
- Are you tired?
- Are you angry about something that's happened before this?
- Have you eaten today?
- Is there anything you're afraid of?
- Once whatever it was went wrong, what were your thoughts, images or feelings?
- Taking the time out to listen to yourself as somebody who cares about you, what do you think now?
- What do you need and how can you give that to yourself?
- Sometimes it's good just to write things out without really thinking about them and then going back fifteen minutes later to underline the feelings words, as sometimes it's hard to connect with what we actually do feel, perhaps preferring the power of anger over, e.g. fear or hurt.

2. When you're worried, breathe. Practise breathing in and out deeply so that the breathing takes all of your attention for a while.
3. Remember to laugh; it's good for the soul.
4. Progress not perfection!
5. Sometimes it's better to live sorry than say sorry. Living amends mean that you change your behaviour not to gain recognition, but to feel at peace with yourself. Be the you you want to be.
6. Step 10: this is a step in the twelve-step process and it's a good discipline to have in your life:
   - Write briefly about your day each day.
   - Notice any conflicts or difficulties and what they brought up for you. Are there any old behaviours you need to take responsibility for?

- o Do you understand what happened – do you need to make any amends?
- o Notice what you did well and if these are consciously new ways of responding.
- o Note your feelings (sometimes these can be underlined from what you've written about your day) and consider what you need.
- o HALT is hungry, angry, lonely, tired – don't let it happen!
- o Share this with someone, and be open to brief feedback, though you can also ask that this is respected as your process and that you're not inviting rescue, just a witness.
- o Note something you feel grateful for.

Although this book does not provide a panacea for all ills, it can equip you with tools that may make things easier and I encourage you, irrespective of whether you get the immediate response that you want, to continue in some of the approaches and behaviours that I have outlined so that you can be a consistent, respectful and loving presence in your children's lives.

If this book helps you to have one less argument, say one less thing that you regret and allows you to feel close to your children even as they pull into their independence, and rightfully so, then it's worth it.

Happiness

'Strive to be happy'. The final line of Max Ehrmann's poem, 'Desiderata', these four simple words have made me think about my attitude to happiness as much as some of the most painful lessons I have learned. How this simple statement has fascinated me for nearly thirty years. I have learned that happiness is not my birthright, but is instead something I can earn, even strive for. 'Strive' – what does that mean? The hardest working verb in the English dictionary and a long way from sitting around and waiting for happiness to fall into my lap. And what does 'happy' mean in this context? And why am I not entitled to it? In the Fellowship, we call it compare and despair.

My attempts to control my unhappiness by making big gestures didn't work, I still felt angry and thwarted, hard done by, my experience of happiness in direct correlation to physical outcomes. Almost as if I had a codependent relationship with my own recovery.

Soon I began to notice how my behaviour, my response to things that happened, affected how happy I felt. I realised that somehow if I let go of the outcome I could still experience a sense of joy, of uplift and of possibility, of gratitude and of life as long as I was connected to myself curiously and with compassion. As long as I was connected to everyone else. Somehow instead of being a victim of circumstance, I started to realise that I was able to be happy anyway, no matter what. Instead of engaging in conflict, I decided to focus on developing a curiosity around how I felt in relation to others, in relation to what happened in my life.

I noted my feelings of rage and hurt and rejoiced simply in my own connection with my consciousness, with me knowing me. I was increasingly proud of my courage to grow and learn. I was surprised at my willingness to hear, I laughed aloud at my second nature that sought to reinstate the denial that had shielded me from the nourishing truth even when I thought I had thrown it out. So I dispensed with it again and again, daily clearing my side of the street. I was stubborn! I accepted with great joy my place as a grain of sand on a big beach of life, perfectly shaped to fit, and no more or less than anyone else. I accepted HP (a higher power) into my life, relieved to only have to manage what I could, my own behaviour born of my thoughts and feelings – what a relief. I felt held, part of, good enough, curious and most importantly happy as that gave me the willingness to keep taking the next step.

Today, I remain as affected by life's ups and downs as anyone else and I continue to have my share of conflict, sickness, betrayal and loss darkening my landscape. But I must admit that even within some very painful experiences, I have found that I can still connect with others, I can surrender to help, I can still grow in love and despite those times of darkness, deep within I do feel happiness. If a parent is unhappy or lonely, the child will feel it. If the parent has unresolved trauma, the child is at a high risk of holding it for them. If the parent doesn't manage these difficult feelings in a healthy way, the child will begin to carry them for them. Teaching a child that happiness can co-exist with sadness is the kind of happiness I am talking about. The kind that doesn't invite rescue, it invites fellowship.

Actions:
- Smile at someone; smile with someone.
- Sing out loud and dance.
- Play music from your youth.
- Do something kind for someone else without telling them.
- Give yourself an affirmation each day, in the mirror if you can.
- Write down ten things you are grateful for every day and include things like seeing a small flower grow through cracks in cement that confirms anything is possible.
- Believe that whatever you learn stays in the bank for tomorrow.
- Be curious and don't take offence.
- Remember to listen.
- Remember to play.
- Remember to be still.

Set yourself free: you only live once, so be brave and make your life yours!

12

ON THE COUCH

A few genuine questions asked by real parents

How do I talk about drugs to my children?

A: It can be difficult to talk to your offspring about drugs, often because you want them to take on your point of view and because if they are teenagers they will surely be hell-bent on defying you. Also some parents take drugs themselves so feel they are unable to tell their children not to, and some parents have little experience of drugs and so feel very out of their depth on the subject. I think what's important is acknowledging that drugs are very present in our culture and very available to our teen population. Therefore not talking about them is, in my view, negligent. I have met many parents who, in anticipation of my view that their teenager is taking drugs, will seek to shut me down by telling me at a social event that they know what I'm going to say, that I believe their child is taking drugs, but they know they're not. That parent will then go on to describe how their child had slept for days and days after returning from a festival, how moody they had been and withdrawn. It's all I can do to stop my jaw from hitting the floor at the extent of their denial. But as several other parents have told me, if they do acknowledge their child is taking drugs then surely they're obliged to do something about it. This is a head-in-the-sand approach that many parents later regret as they missed the opportunity of early intervention.

I think it is vital to talk to your children about drugs, read about what drugs are out there, their effects and so forth, but also don't expect yourself to know all of this information because it's probably just not your scene. What you do know is that drugs exist in multiple forms, causing multiple effects and that the teenage population is at high risk for experimentation and self-medication. Focusing on why somebody uses something (to medicate anxiety, to feel more confident, to let go, to feel good, to belong) and gently seeking to discover if there is a way to help resolve that, while inviting them to really consider the consequences and how they might take responsibility for their own decisions, is a viable way forward.

What do I do if my child asks me if I have tried drugs?

A: This is a really common question and the harsh reality is that rarely is the child actually interested in what happened to you when you were growing up, except perhaps to justify their own behaviour or plans, or to find out how much you know. What I suggest to parents is that the question you want to ask in return is something along the lines of 'I'm more than happy to talk to you about my own experiences growing up, but why are you asking me that now?' You want to know exactly that. Why is this information relevant to your child today? Have they had a drugs talk at school or a PSHE presentation that brought that question up? Maybe it's a sign of their exposure to drugs in their social circle and they're beginning to think about what that means in real terms. Certainly, when I go and talk in schools, the first thing I do as I look at the sea of uniform that stretches out in front of me is to convert that conforming school child into a Saturday night teenager, because that's the person I'm trying to talk to. It's very different making a decision about taking drugs when you're at school or having a conversation at home with your mum or dad, than it is when you're at a party or a gathering.

Test it out: a few days after the initial question make yourself and your teenager a cup of tea and go into their room where they will inevitably be sitting in front of their TV or computer screen, on their mobile and with earphones in while doing their homework. Sit down next to them and, over tea, settle in to tell them about your childhood experiences. Watch the curtain of irritation fall across their face and wake up to the fact of self-centred youth. Whatever it is they want to know, it is for their own ends. If you answer that question in the moment of asking, you have no idea where it is coming from and where your answer will have gone, its impact. Box clever.

What do I do if I believe my son or daughter is taking drugs?

A: This is the worst nightmare of most parents: it takes many out of their comfort zone, and leaves them very scared so that they either bury their heads in the sand or overreact. Neither approach will work. The first step is to take responsibility for the reality that in my view most teens will have subjective experience of drugs by the time they are sixteen – and what I mean by that is that they won't necessarily have used them but they will have come across them in their social circle. You have to decide as a parent where you stand with this and why. You have to think about what it is you're prepared to accept and where the line is drawn because any teen will overstep that line as a matter of principle. So you need to think about drugs as a category, but you also need to think about each individual drug in the same way that the government will grade them in classes and decide if you have any tolerance for your child to experiment with any drug at all, or not. I suggest you do the research so that the position you take is backed up by understanding, showing you are taking the time to learn. I will add this final thought, because we have all been teenagers: are you sure that if you were a teenager today that you wouldn't be doing what your child may be doing? It's so easy to point the finger from a position of age and experience and, in that moment, forget the heady delight of feeling young and invincible, which is to be celebrated, but also carefully contained. Whatever your decision, make sure you let them know you're worried, keep an eye on them to see if they lose interest in other things in their life or their self-care, as if the drugs are taking over, and remind them that drugs don't fix emotional problems. Stay connected.

What is the right age to introduce my child to alcohol? My husband and I disagree.

A: First, I should say that there is no 'right age' to 'introduce your child to alcohol' as it doesn't have to be your job! But I am often asked what my views are about alcohol and children, and whether I believe that it is important to introduce them to alcohol from a young age, somehow normalising it around meal times, for example, instead of making it seem prohibitive, which we all know can create an unnatural level of curiosity and rebellion. There is a second school of thought that suggests that doing exactly this creates a taste for alcohol and that introducing alcohol when the child is old enough to properly consider its impact is the more responsible approach.

As with many conflicting points of view, both approaches have valid pros and cons, so I think each parent should view not only their child or children, but the culture that they represent, through modelled behaviour. As your children hit the teen years, they are likely to start experimenting with alcohol and they will have their experiences where they get very drunk, where they're sick, when they do things that they regret. They will want to 'pre' before a party (in other words get tipsy or drunk before they go), they will want to take a bottle to the party and they don't want you to get in the way. You need to make your mind up about where you stand before this moment comes so that you can be consistent and transparent around your rules as they will be under attack. I personally do not think a teenager should be drinking spirits, certainly not under eighteen years old, so wouldn't send them to a party with a quart of vodka. I'd add that it is in my experience foolhardy to believe that by giving your child a decent bottle of wine that you save them the ill health of the cheap stuff, as they will do both. Teens will play brinkmanship so that they push against the rules and test out your boundaries, and alcohol is often the playground on which this is acted out.

My son wants to drink less when he goes out but he doesn't know if he can. Do you have any tips to help him stay sober – or to drink less – when going out?

A: First, I suggest he honestly establishes why he wants to cut down or stop. Maybe get him to answer the following questions – warning signs to help motivate him:

- Are you sleeping badly and having nightmares, easily woken or having night sweats?
- Is your mood very up and down?
- Do you feel very demotivated or that you can't be bothered?
- Are you excessively irritable?
- Are you prone to not feeling good enough around family, children and friends?
- Do you feel very misunderstood and overlooked?
- Do you feel as if your face just doesn't fit?
- Are you craving a drink? The thought flickers in and out of your mind as if suggesting it will fix how you feel.
- Do you need to drink to function?
- Are you drinking to get rid of physical symptoms like headaches, sweats, shakes?
- Do you decide not to drink and then find yourself drinking?

If he has answered 'yes' to three or more of the above he should really consider addressing his alcohol dependence. Here are a few suggestions as to how to cut down. I hope it helps!

- Write down why you want to cut back.
- Write down how many drinks you are going to have and see if you can stick to it.
- Get support in the social group you'll be with when you're tempted.

- Try finding other ways to deal with stress (see Chapter 1 on anxiety, depression and stress).
- Don't do any pre-drinking.
- Eat well before you go out – carbs help soak up the alcohol, slowing down its effect.
- Try alternating between a glass of water and the alcoholic drink. This will also reduce the physical symptoms caused by dehydration.
- Decide what you're going to drink in advance and see if you can stick to it.
- Notice what makes you want to drink. Is it feeling left out, wanting to let go more or wanting to be more drunk? This will tell you what you need to work on if you want to stop. If alcohol does a job for you, you want to make it redundant.
- The next morning notice how you feel. Did you have a good night without the ill effects? Then, surely that's worth it!

My daughter wants to go to the festivals after her GCSEs and I'm worried but everyone else is going so I can't really say no! Help!

A: Festivals have become a teenage rite of passage especially following the intensity and stress of exams. How easy it is to agree to something to get through the exams and then regret it. Plan in advance so that you know which festivals you are prepared to let your teen attend and who they might go with. Do your research, look at the press reports and talk to your teen about it.

At festivals, no matter how much patting down there is at the gate, drugs will find a way in and strangely many teens tell me that it's harder to get alcohol than it is drugs at many of the UK festivals because that is better policed. I'm often told that just inside the gate, there are people waiting who mutter under their breath offers of pills or powders or weed for just a few pounds. As I'm sure you can imagine, if this goes on over the day or days of the festival, eventually many teens will relent and experiment.

The most powerful prevention is good self-esteem because if somebody cares about themselves they are unlikely to harm themselves. But even in the case of somebody who has a strong sense of worth, in the teen years they may be tempted to experiment and of course sometimes accidents happen. And both dangers need attention. No drug is safe, but this won't stop teens experimenting. Some festivals have locations drug testing to check the drug is what it claims to be. This is a valuable step towards minimising the risk of 'dirty drugs'. The self-esteem issue is longer term and more complex. However, if your child is determined to try and experiment with drugs and alcohol and expose themselves potentially to risky behaviours and unprotected sex then I believe they need to be informed. In that way they can become more responsible for the choices they make in their lives for which they will pay the consequences. Thus as a parent, we have this mixed message: I prefer you didn't try drugs or get out of hand on alcohol. However, if you are determined to experiment or to drink to excess here a few thoughts you should consider:

1. There is no such thing as using drugs safely.
2. Drugs, and certainly the ones we are talking about here, are illegal, and if they're not (i.e. prescription drugs being used for recreational purposes) their application in recreational use might be illegal.
3. Obtaining drugs for a friend is called supplying or dealing and has legal consequences.
4. If you are already taking prescription medication, or suffer from a physical or mental health condition, you should seriously reconsider the wisdom of choosing to experiment with drugs.
5. Never mix your drugs (poly-drug use); mixing drugs or alcohol with other drugs can cause an unpredictable reaction.
6. Be careful not to overhydrate as drinking too much water can be lethal too.

7. Step out of the environment regularly to allow yourself to cool down and recalibrate as naturally as possible, but go with a friend.

8. Do not isolate yourself or go off on your own, as you may become disorientated, or identified as a target. Stay with your friends.

9. Before you go out or go to a festival make sure you know who your 'safe people' are and make the commitment to be there for one another. It is often hard to decide who that person is when you are drug- or alcohol-affected, or in trouble in some way.

10. Do not hesitate to go to the first aid tent or call an ambulance if somebody is suffering the ill effects of drug and alcohol use. Being worried about getting busted is no excuse not to call for help if you're out of your depth.

11. If there is a facility to have your drugs tested so that you know the contents before you take them then use that facility.

12. Drugs have an effect on you mentally and physically. Using them when you are already tired, haven't eaten properly, are anxious, angry or upset about something increases the chances of something going wrong.

13. Really think about what you are doing and consider the price (beyond money) that you may have to pay as a result of the choices you are making. Many people use drugs as a shortcut to a sense of belonging, and often that shortcut backfires. It's important you know that.

14. Risky and sexual behaviour are often part of the experience of getting drunk or wasted. It's worth deciding in advance where your boundaries lie, as figuring that out at the time is likely to be almost impossible. Tell your friends not to let you go off with someone so they have permission to intervene and so that you can stay safe and not cause harm for yourself or anyone else.

Parents sometimes think that in telling their child they tried drugs and then describe a horror story of what happened next might actually put that child off from experimentation. And it might . . . for a while, until they see their friends trying it out. Unfortunately for parents, drugs are everywhere, widely available to all, easy to get hold of, affordable and very much part of the teen scene. For a while, parental advice might be the most influential factor in a child's behaviour, but as those teenage years gather pace, the peer group becomes the bigger influence. Thus, when the child who was previously terrified of even smoking a cigarette sees one of their friends smoking weed or popping a pill and not suffering some horrific consequence, all of your credibility goes out the window. What everybody tends to forget is that we are all on the same side, parents and teens, as we want our kids to have a good time as much as they do, and we want them to be safe. It's worth acknowledging too that rarely do I meet a teenager who is not concerned about their own safety.

If your child is already suffering from emotional difficulties, then it would be worth them seeing a therapist before embarking on a festival summer as they either leave school or finish their GCSEs, because they will be at a greater risk of running into problems. Certainly in my practice, I have worked with families with a troubled teenager who then goes to the festival knowing exactly what will or won't be tolerated. After each event, we have a session to work through their experiences, and they are also held accountable and drug-tested. It's a priceless opportunity to learn and grow in a real-life setting

I have addiction in my family – when do I tell my child?

A: You'll notice I have already written an entire chapter on ACoA (see pages 107–28) and the impact of this condition on other members of the family. I find in families where there is an existing condition of addiction that the parents are either hypersensitive to the possibility of their children suffering from the same and so see it in every interaction or they are relieved not to see it at all. I don't think there's any point in arguing between yourselves as parents as to whether your child is or isn't in the early stages of addiction but I do think that a) respectful boundaries will do no harm and b) making understanding addiction in its broadest sense a comprehensive part of the child's growing up process will help the child spot the signs earlier. I think it's important that addiction is not represented as a life sentence, or something to be ashamed or fearful of, but rather as something to be aware of, and to respect. I would start in those early years with educating the child about The Core Characteristics™, and about what each emotion is and how to have that feeling in a healthy and contained way. Second, I would make sure that any traumatic or stressful event was properly processed and emotionally filed in a way that it is unlikely to cause future disturbance. If you subscribe to the self-medication hypothesis of addiction as a process of using something outside of yourself to fix how you feel to the detriment of yourself, then prevention is knowing it might happen, knowing where it might happen in yourself and believing that you are caring about yourself enough to make sure it doesn't happen. I don't think addiction is anything to be ashamed of nor do I think it is a badge to be worn with pride. It runs in families and so everyone in that family should know an age-appropriate amount about it and learn how not to let it take hold.

Is addiction a chronic relapsing condition?

A: I included this question because it is so very contentious. Almost everybody I know who works in the field or in recovery from addiction believes that addiction is indeed a chronic relapsing condition. Once the pattern of self-medication has been firmly established in relation to uncomfortable feelings, trauma and pain it is hard enough to give up that self-medication and commit to a pathway of experiencing those feelings. Reintroducing the drug of choice is a high-risk strategy because inevitably the primed response, the earliest memory, is to avoid so given the opportunity and reintroduction it's only a matter of time before the 'drug' takes over again. But then I think about eating disorders, codependency, exercise, shopping, work and sex and love addiction – and we have what are known as process or behavioural addictions whereby the abstinence is not in excluding these substances and behaviours from your life but learning how to include them in a healthy way.

This has always fascinated me as a kind of gold standard of recovery, not the controlled using advocated by harm-minimisation promoters but instead that abstinence is when your 'using' isn't using! When treating an eating disorder, it's important to eat three meals per day with snacks in between for anorexic or bulimic clients. All the other hungry feelings can then be recognised as emotional as you know you have given your body what it needs nutritionally. So often someone with an eating disorder will say 'I feel fat' when they feel they are too much or ashamed, 'I feel full or sick' when they have feelings they can't handle, 'I feel hungry' when they are sad or in fear. Instead of feeling the emotions they will feel something more practical, related to food or appetite, and seek to control the emotion through that. Knowing this allows you to disbelieve the message that you're hungry and explore what's going on instead. The same applies to sex and love, intimacy and attachment disorders, and to work, exercise and shopping. So surely if we catch this condition early enough and attend to the wounds that might otherwise feel intolerable before a self-destructive coping mechanism takes hold, then surely we can elicit a cure? But in order to intervene early I believe we need to be looking at the distortion of The Core Characteristics™ rather than waiting for a manifestation to show itself, because by then neural pathways are established to repress and avoid, the pattern is set and we are too late. Better still to parent in such a way that you avoid the dead end that is addiction by promoting healthy relational patterns from the outset.

My child's a fussy eater, should I worry?

A: There are two parts of this question and both need equal attention. One is the eating pattern of the child, and the other is how does the parent handle their worry.

Most people have a few things that they don't like to eat or drink, and that's OK, but fussy eating can be very difficult for a parent to handle and long-term it's not good for the child. You certainly don't want to make mealtimes a battleground but it's important that the parent remain in charge and the child does what he or she is told so that they learn to eat what's in front of them. Making sure that the food is healthy and balanced means that you know as a parent that you are asking your child to eat something that will provide them with the fuel and nutrients they need to be healthy and well, therefore it is not all about whether they like it or not. Healthy meals should have protein and carbohydrates and vegetables at least twice a day and each portion of category of food should be about the same size as the eater's fist. There is also as little salt and sugar as is possible in today's world. It's important not to let them eat snacks between meals that will reduce their appetite too, because if they are hungry they are more likely to eat. There are lots of techniques that are based around reward and fun and distraction that help a child to overcome their stubbornness and to eat. Again if the family is eating at the same time, including the parent or parents, then the modelled behaviour will also play its part.

The time to worry about fussy eating is when it appears to be a coping mechanism, a way of control, a way of gaining attention so that their eating habits dominate (and that can be negative or positive attention) or when there are visible physical consequences that are cause for concern. There is no doubt that eating disorders are difficult to treat because the drug of choice is quite literally everywhere and there is no such thing as complete abstinence. Recovery is 'controlled using'. Try asking that of an alcoholic! Usually patient, firm and good-natured engagement can help a child overcome their resistance to eating certain foods. But if they trigger the parent into losing their temper, or into tears or to over-worry, then it's likely they will hold onto their 'fussy eating' as a comfort or form of control (in the absence of parental control).

This leads me to my comment about parental worry – as how a parent expresses that worry is vital. No child should have to be responsible for their parent's feelings; even if the parent thinks the child has caused the feelings, those feelings are still the parent's responsibility. Therefore, if as a parent you are worried about your child's eating, get yourself the support and information that you need to address it properly because if all you do is tell or show the child you are worried or worry without any answers you are likely to drive them further into their dysfunctional food use.

How do I stop my child developing an eating disorder?

A: As above, through healthy modelled behaviour, through healthy emotional expression, through holding the boundary which reflects your own behaviour as a parent and through realising that rarely is an eating disorder all about the food, and rarely is an eating disorder about the weight. In my experience, an eating disorder is always about emotions and relationship with self and other. Ways to avoid promoting an eating disorder is to ensure that you provide three meals a day, based on set times, not on how anyone feels. Try not to give food as a comfort nor take it away as a punishment. Introduce healthy eating patterns and tastes in food from the early years so that fruit and vegetables form part of their accepted diet. Avoid sweet things as comfort or rewards, as not only will this promote the pattern in later years, but it also fosters a sweet tooth that can be a precursor to liking alcohol as there is a lot of sugar in alcohol. Instead, help your child to express how they feel and sometimes that's all that's needed. No one can provide a solution to a problem every time, but you can be there and provide support by just listening. Helping your child to accept that emotions are a natural part of life and that they are there to tell you what's going on with you in relation to your environment and the people you interact with will help your child develop curiosity in relation to these emotional messages, rather than a need to escape them – because they will just keep coming! If your child's emotions scare you because you don't feel able to handle them, get some help so that you don't feel deskilled by their process. You might be able to get away with it when they are small but as they get bigger you might wish you had got help sooner.

I've heard about tough love but I don't understand it. Surely, it can't be good to do something that hurts someone you love as a way of helping them? I don't want to deliberately hurt my child. I couldn't.

A: Tough love is a term that is firmly associated with recovery from addiction, and people often ask me what it means and why it's important. Simply put, if you repeatedly soak up the consequences of someone else's behaviour by covering for them, apologising for them, paying their debts, then you are enabling. Tough love is often seen as the opposite so that you remove the cushion, stand back and watch as the consequences hit. But this is not quite right as it represents an all-or-nothing response which is often a signature of trauma itself. It's no good going from rescuing and micromanaging to abandonment. Tough Love is, in my view, an application of firm clear boundaries that do not change according to circumstances and which can be perceived as as tough to deliver as to receive, but crucially they are delivered from a position of love, which means they are often painful for the parent when putting them in place. Thus tough love is as much about the person delivering as the person it is aimed for. Tough love usually means that often you remain in contact but you no longer fix the problem. That you continue to tell the person that you care as you stand back and watch them experience the consequences of their own behaviour.

For many parents I work with, this will involve a few key house rules such as no drugs in the home, no alcohol in the home, no drug- or alcohol-affected behaviour in the home, one (sometimes more) family meal a week, no money, although the parent is willing to pay for therapy / phones / travel cards, and also a warning system of yellow and red cards, after which the teenager may be asked to leave the home. This is almost always the hardest moment because every parent is worried that their child will seriously harm themselves or even die if they get kicked out, and most of the time, the teenager knows this.

I think it's important at any point for parents to feel that they have done absolutely everything they can at every stage. It can be very useful to attend a family group or one of the free fellowships, such as Al-Anon, to gain support to do this.

Tough love must come from a place of self-respect and love. Boundaries are an act of respect and love. Rescue and enabling is undermining self-esteem. Change needs to happen consciously, respectfully, transparently and consistently so that if a dynamic moves from enablement to tough love it's unlikely to happen overnight. This is a marathon not a sprint.

We are divorced and we really don't agree with how to parent – how will this affect my child?

A: Often divorced or separated parents come to me with this issue and they are quick to realise the differences they complain about in terms of parenting are the same themes that caused the marriage to breakdown. As a product of that marriage, the child will have to learn how to navigate the differences of opinion. They can only do this when both parties stop competing and just own their own point of view with respect for the other. Sadly this is rarely how it plays out and more often the child is able to exploit the differences, causing frustration in one or both parents, who then go on to blame each other.

Another aspect of this is that one parent often feels like the 'bad parent' and is annoyed that the enabling behaviour of the one who is perceived to be the 'good parent' makes them more popular with the child. It is exactly this irritation and this competitive energy that allows the split. Whatever the rules of your house are, it's important that you understand where those come from in you and why you want it to be like that in your house. Understanding this and then relaying it to your child or children as a consistent representation of who you are and how you live, irrespective of how the other party lives, will allow your child to know you, and from that place know themselves in relation to you.

Of course, it's frustrating if one parent has more money than the other so the child may have access to screens and other privileges that they don't have with you. If this is the case, it will be your challenge to respect whatever wealth it is you have, in whatever form, and to teach your child to appreciate that as part of what you bring to the relationship.

The negative effect on the child of parents who are resentful towards one another in their differing parenting approaches is that neither home is safe and therefore neither parent is safe, because to agree with one is to disagree with the other. It means the child has no one and is likely to withdraw into themselves and possibly even dissociate from how they feel just in case it causes resentment, by whatever they say about one parent to the other.

Trying to compete with the other parent is likely to give the child too much power: they may perceive you as jealous or mean-spirited instead of as hurt or insecure. Your relationship with your child is so precious and I would suggest you do not let anyone or anything poison that bond, so you need to stay focused on you, rather than distracted by the information about your ex-partner. You may find it is your own resentment of your ex-partner that plays out via your relationship with your child: if that is the case, it may be worth your while seeing a therapist, alongside doing some of the worksheets in this book to clear yourself of that toxic thinking. As they say in the fellowships, AA and NA, etc., of which I am a huge and grateful fan: 'what you think of me is not my business'.

Don't let anyone stop you from being the parent you want to be. Never believe you're doing this for your children alone, recognise the pay-off to yourself as you put your head on your pillow at night and feel good enough to sleep soundly and guilt-free.

Is my child addicted to technology?

How can I get my son daughter off his/her phone/ PlayStation/Xbox?

Technology is ruining our lives – help!

A: Technology is here to stay – fact! In my view, we are behind the curve in terms of understanding the effect it's having on us all, the extent of its potential and its influence and in terms of how to manage it. What I'm seeing in my work in schools and at my clinic is the beginnings of an epidemic, and on the ground the parents are ill-equipped to handle it.

This deserves a book in its own right because as a subject it is hugely relevant, greatly undiscussed in a useful way and expansive, with multiple applications that extend into behaviour, human interaction, relationships, communication, development of identity and self-respect, work ethics and accessing potential and human evolution. Technology is affecting every family in the country via smartphones, gaming devices, social media, live streaming and so on, providing, at best, entertainment and interconnection where the world becomes small and, at worst, the very opposite: isolation, avoidance of human interaction, anxiety and depression and an inability to cope with everyday life because the world has become the device.

A long-standing alcoholism cliché applies: the man takes a drink; the drink takes a drink; the drink takes the man. It is vital that we get across the use of technology so that we are in charge of it, we are bigger than it, and it does not control us.

The arguments that I hear about technology use are raging behind closed doors across the country every day, causing damage to the very roots of human relationships – family. The teenager or the child whose technology use means that their need for that device dominates the family home, whether that's not being able to sleep without the iPad, or concentrate without a phone, throwing a tantrum when it gets taken away so that the only way to stop the tantrum is to give it back, being attached to the smart phone to the exclusion of any meaningful interaction with the family, withdrawing to the bedroom for hours on end to engage in gaming . . . Woe betide the parent who tries to intervene because the addicted teenager will fight back.

I hear about sexting as if it were normal; I hear about online bullying as commonplace; I hear of dependence on 'likes' and the crushing blows of any negative comment or trolling; I hear about the hours and days and months spent lost in a virtual world; I note the increased anxiousness and depressive symptoms that seem aligned with excessive screen use and I regret how few clinicians or GPs think to ask the client about this as they do their assessment around a mood disorder, so it often goes unnoticed when it just might be a cause.

What to do? Ask yourself this: have I taught my child to dissociate / numb out by using screens? Cast your mind back to when they were very young and you wanted them to be quiet so that you could get on with some daily chore or maybe simply to have time to yourself. Did you sit them in front of the screen, using it as a babysitter? If so, you may well have taught them that that's what screens are for. Knowing this is not to appoint blame but rather it is to include you in the dialogue that must follow, whereby both of you have fallen foul of something much bigger and stronger than you.

Some simple recommendations for you to consider:

1. No child should possess his or her technology before the age of seven. They can use the family technology but it doesn't belong to them; they will not have the same right of entitlement that can reinforce the tantrum.

2. Be very clear when you let that child use the technology how long they're allowed to go on for and if the child is under seven, it should be no longer than half an hour at any given time.

3. After the technology use, do something active.

4. Between seven and eleven, children need to learn to manage access to technology so that by the time they go to secondary school they can handle having a phone, which most parents want their child to have as a point of contact / safety so these years are the training ground. Prepare yourself for a battle.

5. Between eleven and fifteen, you should have access to all of their accounts but you must treat them with respect. These ideas and boundaries assume the parent to be a responsible adult, not overanxious or over-controlling nor an active addict of any kind, and this is probably unrealistic, so please take my suggestions as guidelines and apply them with as much self-knowledge as you have when you intervene on somebody's technology use. I believe you are interrupting a mainline connection akin to crack addiction; your child will be wired, charged and hyper-stimulated and, as a result, their behaviour

and language will reflect this. If you have given them that technology or permission to use that technology, you have to be able to handle the fallout so that you do not overreact to what I consider to be the inevitable instant withdrawal. When most kids come off their game/phone/social media, etc. and are in withdrawal, it's vital the parent does not get triggered into retaliating with shouting/abuse/physical behaviours, but stays calm so that the child can tune in to how they feel as a result of their tech use, not of how their parent is. This is how they will learn.

What's the point of therapy? How can just talking help?

A: It still amazes me that the simplicity of therapy works, but it just does. The miracle really does happen. Talking to someone who isn't involved means you can say whatever you want and once you've said it, you can change your mind. It's not like talking to a friend who holds on to the information and you end up building a story that can trap you. In therapy, it is confidential and completely non-judgemental, so you can empty your head of all the thoughts and experiences you've kept inside for fear of being thought mad, being misunderstood, offending someone or that someone will think badly of you, without threat. Then you can begin to sift through all the stories and reactions and relationships and feelings and see what's what. Discovering themes can usefully inform you of what's important to you and then you can work to connect it up to past or childhood experience so you understand why. Good therapy allows you to become conscious and compassionate of what has happened to you in your life in such a way that it delivers you a choice so you can be the you that you want to be. While we are not conscious of it, so much of our behaviour is automatic as a result of our formative experience.

Therapy for addiction

- Find a safe place with a therapist you connect with.
- Commit to ten sessions minimum.
- Achieve abstinence as a priority.
- Create boundaries and make relapse difficult.
- Work through what it is that makes your addiction so attractive to you, the thoughts and feelings that drive you can be dismantled and the charge neutralised.
- Maintain your well-being and learn how not to invite the triggers back into your life.
- Find people who are in the same position as you and stick with the winners (try the fellowship meetings).

I am so scared of taking my daughter to a therapist as I think I'll lose her even more. How do I find a good one?

A: I'll deal with the simple part of that question first! There are three recommended routes to finding a good therapist: i) word of mouth – if someone you know has had a good experience, it has worked and they have enjoyed it (yes that's possible!), then go and see that therapist, if not to stay with them, but for an assessment and a referral. Good people tend to know good people; ii) through your GP or another health professional; and iii) through the accredited websites like www.bacp.co.uk or www.emdr.com.

Before committing to a series of sessions, meet the therapist and see if you'd be likely to stick with them, even if they are telling you something you don't want to hear. Once you have decided to commit, then do it. Go every week for a few weeks and months to get connected and then discuss your attendance and listen to advice. Lots of people say they decided not to continue to go because they had nothing they wanted to say, but in my experience that's often when the magic happens!

A parent taking your child to see a therapist is extremely brave and I applaud you. Not only will you feel self-conscious as if you are the one who caused the problem, but also you are probably feeling regret that you couldn't solve it. But any decent therapist will know this, many have walked the walk you are about to take and will have genuine compassion for you in bringing your child to find help. Decent therapy respects the family relationship and simply facilitates a discussion that should then translate outside the therapy room, though sometimes this is in behaviour not a big conversation. No, you shouldn't share a therapist with your child. Yes, they need to have privacy or they won't be honest. Yes, you should know if your child (under sixteen) is or isn't attending. Yes, it's OK to ask for a joint session with a therapist your child's therapist can recommend. No, it's not OK to quiz your child (no matter how passively) after their session. Yes, it's normal to feel blamed for a while, but it's probably your own blame and regret and nothing that your child or their therapist is saying. Remember that.

For as long as you feel guilt, your child doesn't have to take responsibility. Take the risk to go the distance and dig deep, note your guilt, learn from it and then let it go. Make your apologies through living change and show that change can happen. Be the parent you want to be, and don't let anyone get in your way – least of all your children!

FEELINGS

As follows are a series of words to help you describe angry, sad, fearful or ashamed feelings – these are the ones that often cause the most trouble. The more specific you can be, the more curious, the better you can represent yourself.

Angry feelings:

Annoyed	Grumpy	Seething
Aggravated	Hateful	Spiteful
Belligerent	Hostile	Violent
Bitter	Impatient	Worked up
Boiling over	Incandescent	
Bristling	Incensed	
Cold	Infuriated	
Contempt	Intolerant	
Cranky	Irritated	
Cross	Livid	
Disappointed	Mad	
Exasperated	Offended	
Fed up	Outraged	
Frustrated	Rageful	
Fuming	Resentful	
Furious	Sarcastic	

Fear feelings:

Afraid	Edgy	Petrified
Alarmed	Fearful	Self-doubting
Anxious	Fidgety	Shaky
Apprehensive	Hesitant	Shocked
Awry	Indecisive	Startled
Cautious	Insecure	Terror
Concerned	Intimidated	Uneasy
Disconcerted	Jumpy	Vigilant
Distrusting	Nervous	Watchful
Dread	Panic	Worried

Sad feelings:

Bleak	Gloomy	Mournful
Dejected	Grief	Regretful
Depressed	Heart-broken	Sad
Despair	Heavy-hearted	Sorrowful
Down	Hopeless	Weepy
Forlorn	Low	Wistful

Shame and guilt feelings:

Ashamed	Flushed	Rueful
Awkward	Flustered	Self-conscious
Contrite	Humiliated	Sheepish
Culpable	Mortified	Sorry
Degraded	Remorseful	Withdrawn
Disgraced	Reproachful	Wrong
Embarrassed	Reticent	

THE ESSENTIALS

Included here are further details and explanations of terms that I have used throughout the book as well as other related terms you might find helpful.

ACoA

Adult Child of the Alcoholic; recognition that growing up in an environment of alcoholism or in a dysfunctional family causes mental health and relationship difficulties.

Basics of Prevention

- Recognise every emotion and be able to name it
- Focus on teaching self-regulation around The Core Characteristics™ encouraging a healthy self-interest (curiosity) and self-care (personal responsibility)
- Teach respect for both boundaries and rules (consistency)
- Model a pattern of healthy helping where there is a shoulder-to-shoulder approach (support) rather than a shaming or rescuing one (control)
- Encourage assertiveness over aggression (stand up for myself vs stand up to you)
- Affirm and criticise based on principles not personalities. For example, 'that took courage to do what you did' or 'I find your behaviour unacceptable' rather than 'you are difficult'

- Inspire interest in e.g. school as a microcosm of life. What's this all about? Involve the child in thinking about this and finding out who they are within it
  - Teach perspective, just for today, so that they learn that this too, whatever it is, will pass (resilience)
  - Teaching from a position of well-being and good self-care yourself is essential, for it is only when I know that I matter can I show you that it's right to believe that you do
  - Promote asking for help if you need it – as someone wise once said, 'you can't chew meat with one tooth!'
  - Realise that you are involved in any interaction that you are in and that there is no such thing as an objective view, so be open around your curiosity as to what is your part and encourage the same in your child (this can alleviate the fear of being to blame)
  - Enjoy!

Bottom and Top lines

Another way of referring to abstinence for a behaviour, so that the bottom line behaviour is specific and one that the person seeking abstinence will avoid. Top lines are conscious goals that people set around what they do want to include.

BUC(k)ET

The Five Core Social Motives as identified by Susan Fiske in her book *Social Beings* (2009) are as follows: Belonging, Understanding, Controlling, Enhancing Self and Trusting (BUC(k)ET). Belonging drives all the other core social motives, which combined facilitate effective functioning in social groups.

DSM-5

The *Diagnostic and Statistical Manual of Mental Disorders* (5th edn) is the 2013 update to the *Diagnostic and Statistical Manual of Mental Disorders* (1952), the taxonomic and diagnostic tool published by the American Psychiatric Association.

EMDR: Eye Movement Desensitisation Regulation

A form of trauma therapy that works through bilateral stimulation (stimulating both sides of the brain) to access the trauma memory and process the information in a way that allows it to be worked through and the trauma symptoms to dissipate. No one can change what has happened to you, but you can change how you store or file it in your memory and your body.

Enmeshment

This is when people become so close that the boundaries between them become blurred, and you cannot tell whose feelings are whose, and sometimes lose individual identity, as they are so closely intertwined

FOMO

Fear of Missing Out – a term that has come with the digital age and prompted by social media posts, FOMO describes an anxiety that an exciting or interesting event may currently be happening elsewhere.

God

Please don't be put off by the 'God' word. Too many use this as an excuse not to go to twelve-step meetings or be part of the programme (see page 227). It is a fellowship that was born of Christian principles, but the simple action was how one drunk helped another to get and stay sober. Within the fellowship most people would say that 'God is for people who don't want to go to hell, and spirituality is for those who have been there'. The 12 steps are most definitely a spiritual programme. God can mean whatever you need it to mean – some say 'Group of Drunks', others refer to the power of nature, some to the fellowship or their therapeutic group. All it really means is that you surrender to help, not to one person as a guru, but to a spiritual principle that allows you to be you, no better or worse than anyone else, in the best way you can be. Some people in recovery experience a spiritual awakening as a result of the work they do and others do find God in the traditional sense, but it is not a prerequisite.

Karpman's Drama Triangle

A relational pattern (a triangle) of roles which circulate around blame and shame. The three roles are those of a persecutor, a victim and a rescuer. Most people recognise themselves in one or two of these roles but if you are one you are all three. The **persecutor** experiences power and a self-righteous view that accuses. The **victim** has a role with no personal responsibility prone to feeling hopeless and helpless. The **rescuer** is the moral arbiter, the one with answers and urgent to help. The rescuer casts who is the persecutor and victim by where they place their support and is often completely unaware of this influence as they more often see themselves as entering a conflict to sort it out not reinforce it. The triangle is not static and you can enter as a rescuer, find yourself persecuting and then end up in victim. You can do it with others or all on your own. Dr Karpman's book *A Game Free Life* is also well worth a read.

Living Amend

Connected to the twelve-step fellowship where amends form part of the recovery programme (steps 8 and 9), a living amend is an apology applied by changed behaviour so that instead of apologising, you change your behaviour to show your sincerity and learning. It is also a way of addressing regret through changed behaviour which may not even be towards the person who was part of the original experience, but for your own self-respect.

Maslow's Eight Basic Needs

Abraham Maslow conceptualised the eight basic needs (Maslow, 1943), which he introduced as: physiological (basic self-care facilitates balanced mood), safety, belonging, self-esteem, cognitive (to learn, explore, discover and create), aesthetic, self-actualisation (striving) and self-transcendence (spiritual). He illustrated these as a triangle, in the order as written here, with each providing a foundation for the next, to allow achievement of the top of the triangle, transcendence.

Meetings

There are mixed meetings, women's and men's meetings, LGBT meetings, themed meetings and open and closed meetings. An 'open meeting' is for anyone interested and 'closed' is for those who identify as an addict of that fellowship. The goal is to be sober (for whichever fellowship), 'just for today'. If you're a newcomer, try to go early, sit at the front and talk to people.

PTSD

Post-Traumatic Stress Disorder is a disorder that presents as anxiousness or depression and is caused by the experience of a very stressful or frightening incident that was not properly processed at the time, leaving unresolved feelings of fear that can in turn cause symptoms such as flashbacks, disturbed sleep and appetite, nightmares, volatile mood and isolation.

Queen Bee

Behaviour of a group of girls who gather around one powerful character to establish themselves in a group that feels safe, reinforcing that sense of safety by criticising others who are not in the group. Usually fuelled by insecurity, these girls can be experienced as bullies by others.

Splitting

A term used to described the difficulty a person has in holding opposing thoughts, feelings and beliefs, like in black and white thinking. It is a common defence mechanism that allows someone to feel certain of another as good/bad, right/wrong with no grey area.

Sponsor

This is someone in the twelve-step fellowship programme who has a couple of years of sobriety under their belt, who has worked the steps themselves, and who is in a position to take a newcomer through them too. The sponsor costs nothing except commitment and gains by giving back. The idea is for the newcomer to approach someone at or after a meeting as a potential sponsor who is the same gender and whose recovery they admire. Once the sponsorship has begun the newcomer should call and meet their sponsor regularly, and follow the suggestions the sponsor makes. This is not a friendship, though after many years of sobriety past sponsors can become friends; it is an arrangement that benefits both parties to consolidate a robust recovery. NB: if someone offers to be your sponsor, ask yourself why, as it's your job as the newcomer to make the approach. Your recovery is yours and every step you take yourself belongs to you: treasure each one!

The Core Characteristics™

A list of human characteristics that I believe are pivotal in the prevention of addiction since if they are overlooked, a vital opportunity of early inter-vention is missed: control (against vulnerability), denial, deceit, fear, shame, compulsion, obsession, projection, expectation, resentment, isolation, self-centredness/self-pity/self-will.

The Five Things™

A way to step off the Drama Triangle (let go of the outcome).

1. Gratitude (if only for noticing what you are doing)
2. Repeat verbatim what the other person said (don't say 'I hear you' as the next word will be 'but', indicating you didn't actually listen with your heart)
3. Acknowledge the wisdom of their point; it probably makes sense that the other person thinks and feels the way they do, maybe you have even set them up by past behaviour; this doesn't mean you have to agree but it does mean you have to listen
4. Offer your perspective; no 'but' or 'however' – instead try saying 'may I tell you how I see it?'
5. Gratitude, not for changing the other person in any way, but for the opportunity of representing yourself with dignity and respect – that's an outcome worth having

The Manifestations of Addiction

In my opinion, there are fifteen common actions that people delegate their emotional process to in order to fix how they feel to the detriment of themselves: drugs, alcohol, food, sex and love, gambling, money, work, exercise, self-harm, nicotine, caffeine, shopping, OCD, screens, codependence.

The Twelve-Step Fellowship Programme (see also 'meetings')

A free global support network that promotes abstinence and recovery by remaining abstinent and working through the 12 Steps (*see below*) with the support of a sponsor. There are 12 step programmes available worldwide for such groups as follows: Alcoholics Anonymous (for alcoholics); Al-Anon (for family members of alcoholics, but increasingly for other addictions too); Al-Ateen (for young people affected by a parent's addiction); Narcotics Anonymous (for those addicted to drugs); Gamblers Anonymous; Cocaine Anonymous; Overeaters Anonymous (the main eating disorder fellowship); ABA (Anorexics and Bulimics Anonymous); SLAA (Sex and Love Addicts Anonymous); SAA (Sex Addicts Anonymous); ACA (Adult Children of Alcoholics and Dysfunctional Families), DA (Debtors Anonymous); CoDA (Codependents Anonymous); UA (Underearners Anonymous); OCA (Obsessive Compulsive Anonymous).

The Twelve Steps

Twelve steps that your sponsor (see related entry above) will take you through to complete your recovery programme.

1. We admitted we were powerless over alcohol – that our lives had become unmanageable [*basically: my way didn't work*]
2. Came to believe that a Power greater than ourselves could restore us to sanity [*but I kept trying the same thing expecting a different result*]
3. Made a decision to turn our will and our lives over to the care of God as we understood Him [*realised I couldn't do this on my own so let others, or something greater than me, in to help*]
4. Made a searching and fearless moral inventory of ourselves [*looked at my part in my pain and resentment, and noted the themes, acknowledging that I am the common denominator in my experiences*]
5. Admitted to God, to ourselves and to another human being the exact nature of our wrongs [*got honest with others*]
6. Were entirely ready to have God remove all these defects of character [*decided to change and let go*]
7. Humbly asked Him to remove our shortcomings [*sincerely sought to let go of how I was primed to see the world – as per my step 4*]
8. Made a list of all persons we had harmed, and became willing to make amends to them all [*just that*]
9. Made direct amends to such people wherever possible, except when to do so would injure them or others [*vital to note the*

second part of this sentence – don't do more harm under the banner of getting honest]

10. Continued to take personal inventory and when we were wrong promptly admitted it [*mini steps 4 & 9 every day*]

11. Sought through prayer and meditation to improve our conscious contact with God as we understood Him, praying only for knowledge of His will for us and the power to carry that out [*prayer and meditation are an important part of this daily discipline as otherwise we react instead of responding. We need to learn how to practise peaceful reflection*]

12. Having had a spiritual awakening as the result of these steps, we tried to carry this message to alcoholics and to practise these principles in all our affairs [*tell others that it works if you work it; show them the way*]

Transactional Analysis

A widely recognised form of modern psychology and developed by Eric Berne in the 1960s. TA is based on the concept that everyone has three ego states, parent, adult and child, and that to better understand and respond to these allows personal growth and can improve relationships.

Trolling

This is when someone seeks to upset or cause emotional hurt by posting messages that are personal or inflammatory on social media sites (a form of bullying).

Virtual Communication

A technique to ensure a person understands from the very start that no one communicates in the virtual medium to you as a person, but to you as someone who is one step removed. This allows a different form of expression that might feel more intimate when positive or like a personal attack when negative as the usual forms of self-regulation are not present in the interaction, like non-verbal cues, facial expression and body language. Helping your child appreciate this will help them to become more resilient in their virtual communication with others. No one thinks of the kid in the bedroom on their own receiving the message, they are more aware of their own rude or unpleasant message as if it was daring or witty. Teach your child to turn off their phone early on in the evening, so they are less exposed to the potential of a negative message coming in late at night and support them to talk to you about it, which most will only do if they feel you won't overreact. Stay involved.

REFERENCES

Bettelheim, B. 1987. *A Good Enough Parent: A Book on Child-rearing* (1st edn). Vintage Books.

Dayton, T. 2012. *The ACOA Trauma Syndrome: The Impact of Childhood Pain on Adult Relationships*. Deerfield Beach, FL: Health Communications.

Fiske, S.T. 2009. *Social Beings: Core Motives in Social Psychology* (2nd edn). Wiley.

Fiske, S.T., and Taylor S.E. 1984. *Social Cognition*. Random House.

Karpman, S. 2014. *A Game Free Life*. Drama Triangle Publications.

Karpman, S. 1968. 'Fairy Tales and Script Drama Analysis'. *Transactional Analysis Bulletin*, 7(26), 39–43.

Kübler-Ross, E. 1997. *On Death and Dying*. Simon & Schuster.

Maslow, A.H. 1943. 'A Theory of Human Motivation'. *Psychological Review*. 50 (4): 370–96.

Middleton-Moz, J., and Dwinell, L. 1986. *After the Tears: Reclaiming the Personal Losses of Childhood*. Deerfield Beach, FL: Health Communications.

Wegscheider-Cruse, S. 1980. *Another Chance: Hope and Health for the Alcoholic Family*. Deerfield Beach, FL: Health Communications.

Winnicott, D.W. 1953. 'Transitional Objects and Transitional Phenomena'. *International Journal of Psychoanalysis*, 34: 89–97.

Woititz, J.G. 1983. *Adult Children of Alcoholics*. Deerfield Beach, FL: Health Communications.

Useful websites

BACP (accredited counselling and psychotherapy website, find a therapist)
www.bacp.co.uk/search/Therapists
EMDR
www.emdr.com
Frank
www.talktofrank.com
UKCP (accredited counselling and psychotherapy website, find a therapist)
www.psychotherapy.org.uk/find-a-therapist/

Twelve-step anonymous fellowships

Adult Children of Alcoholics and Dysfunctional Families UK (ACA)
www.adultchildrenofalcoholics.co.uk
Al-Anon Family Groups (for the families and friends of alcoholics)
www.al-anonuk.org.uk
Alcoholics Anonymous (AA)
www.alcoholics-anonymous.org.uk
Anorexics and Bulimics Anonymous (ABA)
www.aba12steps.org
Cocaine anonymous (London) (CA)
www.ca-london.org
Codependence Anonymous (CoDA)
www.coda-uk.org
Debtors Anonymous (DA)
www.debtorsanonymous.org.uk
Families Anonymous (FA)
www.famanon.co.uk
Gamblers Anonymous (GA)
www.gamblersanonymous.org.uk
Marijuana Anonymous (MA)
www.marijuana-anonymous.org.uk

Narcotics Anonymous (NA)

  www.ukna.org

Obsessive Compulsive Anonymous (OCA)

  www.obsessivecompulsiveanonymous.org.uk

Overeaters Anonymous (OA) (main eating disorder fellowship)

  www.oagb.org.uk

Sex Addicts Anonymous (SAA)

  www.saauk.info

Sex and Love Addict Anonymous (SLAA)

  www.sla.org.uk

The National Association for Children of Alcoholics (NACoA)

  www.nacoa.org.uk

Underearners Anonymous (UA)

  www.underearnersanonymous.co.uk

INDEX

ACKNOWLEDGEMENTS

I must acknowledge my deepest gratitude to the following people who have played such a significant part in my life, without some of whom I'm not sure I'd be here. In the last few years, I have made some lifelong friends (I hope), and I sincerely thank you. You have taught me about friendship, trust and self-respect and I aim to bring much of what I have learned to this book.

At the top of my list and from the bottom of my heart are my three children, Daniel, Maisie and Tom. I cherish your company and it is a privilege to be a part of your lives. You have transformed me from an owl to a lark so that I get up in the morning and face my day with gratitude. You have taught me how to be a parent that I am happy to be, and I am so very grateful and proud of you, each one of you.

My mother, we laugh that you have given me my best material for this book, but you have also given me the resilience to keep trying and you have never lost faith in me. Your love is tremendous and unwavering and for that I am forever grateful.

Jane Nudd, my oldest and closest friend, with you I can laugh, head in hands, as we reflect on the experiences of our youth. You stood by me as my life fell apart and for the painful steps as I rebuilt it. You have taught me what real friendship is. Thank you for always being so kind and honest with me.

Tony McLellan, without you I would not be here. You saved my life. You then inspired me to follow this journey to become a therapist and you have taught me so much along the way, including how to laugh in the dark times. You mean the world to me.

My Clinical Supervisor and so much more, I trust you, which is not something I do easily and you have my deepest respect. I am eternally grateful for your no-nonsense wisdom, your sense of humour and for believing in me. I am so grateful to have you in my life and at my side.

Simone Barten, you are my friend. You make me laugh and stand beside me in times of difficulty. Thank you for being so passionate about the message in this book, for asking interesting questions and for reminding me that parents need to know!

My team at Charter, you have taken the model I painstakingly developed and put it into practice. Thank you for the faith you have had in me and in my work, and for making it real! You are all stars in your own right: Zoe Aston, Mu'Dita Farrell, Fira Karimova, Lou Perry, Marie Claire Prust, Tanya Refsen, Victoria Smith, your loyalty means the world to me; my friend and accountant Karen Austin Taylor who makes it all feel possible; and the stars of tomorrow Rhiannon Hudd, Victoria Loxton Edwards, Maika Spooner, thank you for all that you do. There are many more too numerous to mention by name, but whose passion and interest has taught me so much.

Michael Rowlands, you are a 'G' (look it up!). I find your passion and respect for my work and for a life in recovery humbling. Thank you for being my friend, you are one of the most generous people I know.

Nick Brown, when we were teenagers you got me home safe. These last two years you have got my children home safely as I worked. Despite your own difficulties, you have been there for me when I really needed the support and you have had the courage to give me challenging feedback which helped me write a better book – brave man! Thank you.

Jadeen Singh, my agent at John Noel, you helped me to take my first steps into the world of television, press and media and made it all seem so possible. Your belief in me and what I do has helped me to believe in me too.

Olivia Morris at Orion Books, whose faith in me and the message I bring has brought this dream of publishing a book to life. Thank you for your editorial input and feedback – it has been invaluable!

My thanks to Salli Anstey, who always finds a way, to Emma Cole of Positive Healing for your kindness and healing, to Rick Leyland for caring, to Sarah Quested and Natalie Chapman for keeping me looking tidy despite my hectic schedule, and to Apsey and your lovely family, who have gone beyond the call of duty to keep me going. Truly one of life's gems.

Finally, to you, my clients and your families, I owe my greatest debt of gratitude, that you might trust me with your most precious people and open up to me about what frightens you or leaves you feeling ashamed. I know how hard it is to get into recovery and am forever in awe of the process, as it does work – you are all living proof. Thank you for surrendering to help, to doing the next right thing and for carrying the message: 'it works if you work it, so work it – you're worth it'. Bank that!

ABOUT THE AUTHOR

Mandy Saligari is an addiction, parenting and relationship expert with a strong media platform. She specialises in individuals and families affected by broad-spectrum addiction and addictive processes. She is a highly respected and established expert – committed to helping people live healthy, happy, addiction-free lives and preventing addiction running through families and society. She is passionate about dispelling the myths surrounding addiction and mental health. Mandy is also committed to regular talks at schools on early intervention, addiction, emotional coping mechanisms and self-esteem. Mandy has three children.